THE COMPLETE BOOK OF ABS

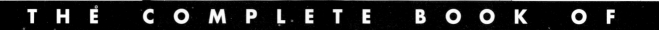

THE COMPLETE BOOK OF

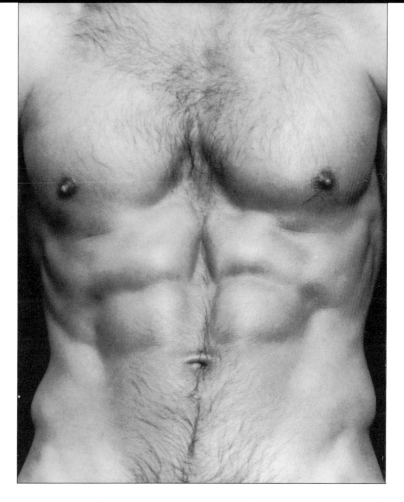

ABs

REVISED AND EXPANDED EDITION

KURT BRUNGARDT

VILLARD BOOKS
NEW YORK

To my mother and grandmother for their support,
no matter what I did,
and to my
brothers and father,
who were my biggest influence in
sports and working out

Since the first edition of *The Complete Book of Abs,* the interest and obsession with ABs has continued to grow: new machines, dozens of articles appear every month, and new diets and supplements continually show up on the scene. I've written two other books, *The Complete Book of Butt and Legs* and *The Complete Book of Shoulders and Arms,* and the media still call primarily to talk about ABs. Our obsession is here to stay.

The purpose of the second edition is to stay updated with this growth and continue to emphasize the basics. By the basics I mean three things necessary to shape and strengthen your ABs: specific AB exercises, cardiovascular work, and a healthy and balanced diet. And you have to be consistent. The second edition re-inforces these principles with new exercises, routines, recipes, and a meal planner to help you organize your eating and workout schedule.

The second edition remains a reference resource packed with information useful to athletes, coaches, personal trainers, and advanced fitness enthusiasts. We have also tried to make this edition more user-friendly. We have simplified the system, added a less-complicated "Get Started Now System," and included a basic weight-training program. The second edition is really for your whole body. It's everything you need to get started on a complete fitness program. Train hard, train smart.

Kurt Brungardt

A C K N O W L E D G M E N T S

I would like to thank Strength Advantage, Inc., for its expertise and guidance through every stage of this book. In particular, I would like to thank Mike and Brett Brungardt for their support.

I would like to thank Bryon and Debbie Holmes for their input and help.

I would like to thank Dave Johnson for his support and proofreading.

I would like to thank Erin O'Hara for almost killing me, but in the long run making me stronger.

I would like to thank all the contributors, strength coaches, and fitness experts who gave time and wisdom to this project—without them it would not exist.

I would like to thank Andrew Brucker for the brilliant photography work he did on the cover and for the exercise photos. Who said artists are hard to work with? It was fun.

And I would like to thank my editor, Doug Stumpf. Doug's vision was the genesis of this book and an essential influence throughout its creation. Doug was a constant source of support, guidance, and patience through every step of the journey. And most important, he made the whole process pleasurable, instead of filled with anxiety.

For the second edition I would like to thank Adam Rothberg for his input and support.

C O N T E N T S

Part Four: The Routines

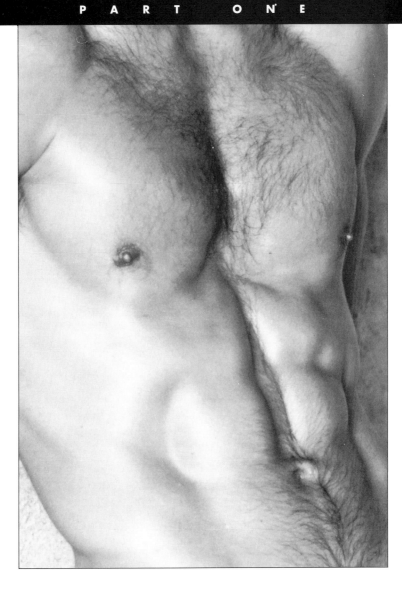

The Foundation

WORLD'S RECORD FOR THE MOST SIT-UPS IN TWENTY-FOUR HOURS?
60,690 by Lou Scripa, 1985

CHAPTER ONE

Working Out: The Truth

by KURT and BRETT BRUNGARDT

Why a Book on ABs Only

Your ABs are the center of your body. They are part of almost every movement you do. They are the core of your strength and power. Every time you lift, bend, twist, shift weight, or balance, power is transferred through your ABs. Strong ABs are essential for good posture and preventing lower-back problems, which makes them a key area in your physical well-being.

The ABs are also the key to physical beauty. Everyone is concerned with having a flat midsection. If you see someone on the beach and his or her ABs are toned, you assume that person's in good shape. And if you see someone with a gut, you assume he or she is out of shape.

Considering their importance, the abdominal muscles have always been shortchanged in exercise books. They are usually given a single chapter with seven or eight exercises and two or three routines. *The Complete Book of ABs* offers over a hundred different exercises and dozens of routines all in one volume.

Most important, this book ties in AB work with sound training principles. It's not as simple as it used to be. To ensure a balanced abdominal workout, you need to do more than get down on the floor and crank out a hundred sit-ups. The ABs are like any other body part. The different areas of the abdomen need to be worked in isolation. You need a large pool of exercises (everyone has personal favorites), so you can create variety in your routines, causing your muscles to continually adapt and improve, giving you the best overall development. In this book, you will find answers to the

AB questions you always wanted to ask. Questions such as: How long and how often should I train? What exercises should I start with? How often should I change my routine? Should I do my exercises in a certain order? How hard should I push myself? Should I work out if I'm sore? Which exercises are most effective for which areas? Are certain exercises dangerous for my lower back? Does my mind play an important role in working out? How should I change my diet to help trim up my ABs?

You will find the answers to these and other questions in this book.

The Truth

The truth is: There are no shortcuts to great ABs. The only way to trim and tone your ABs is through a combination of consistent, focused AB exercises, a disciplined diet, and regular cardiovascular work (running, biking, rowing, etc.). The bright spot in the midst of this harsh reality is that once you accept the truth, it's easy to get what you want. A good plan is half the battle. This book maps out a step-by-step process to help you achieve your goals.

Your part of the bargain is making the commitment. This shouldn't scare or intimidate you. It doesn't mean signing your life away. It means working your ABs five to ten minutes a day, three times a week. But you must do this consistently, making exercise a regular part of your life. It makes no sense to exercise three months and then take a month off. Set realistic goals and then work toward them. The benefits of this small commitment will surprise you. Your muscles will start to firm up, backaches may dissipate, and your posture will improve. Once the workout habit is established, you will naturally want to move on to the next level. Remember: "A journey of a thousand miles starts with a single step."

Myths and Facts

There are many misconceptions surrounding the ABs. There is an absurd history of gimmicks that promise to trim the ABs: plastic suits, suction devices you hook to your vacuum cleaner, waist girdles to wear to the office, and machines that jiggle your belly. Here are some common myths surrounding the ABs.

1. *Sit-ups will make me lose weight around my waist so I look good in a swimsuit.*
Current theory shows that exercise stimulates fat reduction throughout the entire body, not in localized areas. You can't "spot-reduce" specific areas. Tests done on tennis players show their dominant arm (the arm with which they swing the racket) is bigger and has more muscle mass than their inactive arm—*but has the same fat percentage.* Similarly, if you work out your stomach with isolation exercises, that area will get stronger and firmer, but you will not reduce the fat specifically in that area. The new tone will be underneath your fat layers. Only by burning more calories than you take in will you reduce your fat percentage, and this will take place throughout your entire body. Only when you lose the fat will you be able to see the new, defined muscles of your stomach.

2. *If I stop exercising, all my muscle will turn to fat.*
Muscle cannot turn into fat. They are two entirely different molecular structures. If you stop exercising, your muscles will slowly decrease in size. They will not change to fat or anything else. But when you stop working out, you start burning fewer calories and storing more fat. In other words, the muscles shrink and you'll probably gain fat.

3. *If I work out hard and often enough, I can get a stomach like a professional bodybuilder.*
Professional bodybuilders are the exception rather than the rule. They are genetically endowed for this sport, much like someone who is seven feet tall is genetically inclined for basketball. And even bodybuilding champions don't look like Mr. Olympia 365 days a year. They go through strict pre-competition routines that are extreme and may involve questionable health practices. These can include use of steroids, diuretics, extreme low-calorie diets, and extensive and dedicated workouts (up to six hours a day). Extreme diet and dehydration give the "rippled" competition look that is nearly impossible to achieve without such mea-

sures. And this look can be maintained for only short periods of time without severe health risks.

4. *If I do two hundred sit-ups a day, my stomach will be in great shape.*

The traditional sit-up is an exercise that involves other muscles besides the ABs (primarily the hip-flexor muscles). It does not isolate and stress the AB muscles to produce total development. To achieve complete ABs development, you must have a balanced routine that works all the muscles in the abdominal area. And you must work these muscles from a variety of angles.

5. *I'm too old to have a firm stomach.*

Although studies indicate you may lose muscle mass as you become older, you may be able to slow or reverse the process through exercise. There is no reason you cannot improve the strength, flexibility, and overall appearance of your ABs, no matter how old you are. The old adage "Use it or lose it" applies here. Most people lose muscle mass because they stop exercising, not because they're old. They become sedentary. Depending on your present level of fitness, you may be able to add muscle mass. Many dedicated athletes and bodybuilders now in their sixties still have the bodies of thirty-year-olds. You're never too old to receive the health benefits of exercise.

6. *The only way I can burn calories is in aerobics class or on the stationary bike.*

Although cardiovascular work is one of the most efficient ways to burn calories, you burn calories by just existing. You may not receive a digital readout of how many calories you've burned after doing your ABs or lifting weights, but you are burning calories at an increased rate because muscle is an active tissue. The more muscle you have, the more calories you will burn naturally. This doesn't mean you should neglect your cardio training, but rather you should aim for a balance.

7. *My AB workout is really tough. I do a thousand reps a day. It takes me a half hour. And I still don't get the results I want.*

Although there are many variables involved in effec-tive abdominal training, quantity may be the least important. The most important thing is quality. The components that make up quality include: intensity of exercise, proper exercise technique, and following sound training principles. This boils down to doing the right exercise the right way. It means being focused on each and every repetition, feeling every contraction. It does not mean doing your workout on automatic pilot.

8. *For women only: If I do a lot sit-ups, my stomach will get muscular like a man's.*

The possibility of a woman developing large muscle mass is unlikely because women do not produce enough of the hormone (testosterone) and/or enzymes that are primarily responsible for producing muscle enlargement. The look that female bodybuilders attain is the result of extreme training habits like those mentioned in myth number 3. Working your ABs five to ten minutes a day will not give you an overmuscled midsection. It will help you strengthen and tone that area.

9. *If I play a lot of sports, I don't need to work my stomach.*

One of the most important training principles is specificity. Most sports do not specifically train the AB muscles. They do not place sufficient demand on the area to bring about optimal results. Therefore, an AB training regimen is needed to bring about overall development. A sound training program will improve your performance, reduce your potential for injury, and help shape your midsection. If you need proof of this, just go to any softball diamond in the country and look at all the potbellies.

10. *My stomach will never look like a model's. I just don't have the time or the willpower to spend two hours a night in the gym, so why bother?*

Many benefits can be gained from exercise other than a beautiful body; most important, improved health. The latest longevity studies show that doing a little exercise can mean a lot. You don't have to spend hours in the gym to receive important health benefits. Doing a minimum amount of AB work will strengthen your midsection, which will, in turn, improve your posture, support your lower back, decrease chances of injury, and improve your efficiency in everyday movements and activities. In short, it will improve the quality of your life. When you think about it, it's not a bad trade-off for a few minutes of work a day.

11. *Since I'm a woman I need to train my stomach differently.*

When it comes to training your ABs, gender isn't all that important. You need to do the same exercises with the same repetition schemes, you need to eat smart, and do cardiovascular work. The main difference as far as AB work is concerned is where you are genetically predisposed to store fat. Men will store it on their obliques (love handles), women will store it on their lower ABs. It's important to be aware of these problem areas so you don't beat yourself up when your lower ABs lag behind.

The Complete ABs Philosophy

You need a comprehensive program that fits your personal needs. You need a complete abdominal training program that will give you the results you want. The following chapters will give you everything you need to know about training your ABs. You will learn a variety of exercises and routines to train your entire abdominal area, regardless of your fitness level. The concept of complete abdominal training may sound intimidating. You might think you need to hire a personal trainer or be an expert in exercise physiology to use this system. Not true. This book is like having a personal trainer. It breaks down the process step-by-step and educates you along the way.

CHAPTER TWO

Body Basics: Anatomy

by BRETT BRUNGARDT

Four muscle groups make up the abdominal area. These muscles control the movement of the area either independently or in an assisting capacity. The exercises that follow are designed to train these muscles in isolation, working to correct areas of weakness and imbalance. Combination exercises are also included to train two or more muscles at once, producing a synergistic relationship between the muscles that resemble everyday movements.

The following drawings show origin and insertion points. Anatomically speaking, muscles originate at one bone and insert at another. Typically, the origin attaches to the least movable bony part and the insertion attaches to the most movable bony part.

The purpose of this chapter is not to make you an expert in anatomy. You don't have to memorize insertion and origin points. But you should be able to connect the name of each muscle to its location on your body. And you should know the movement function of each muscle: to bend side to side, to twist, to raise and lower the torso, etc. You need this knowledge to aid visualizations and help create the mind-muscle link described in Chapter 4.

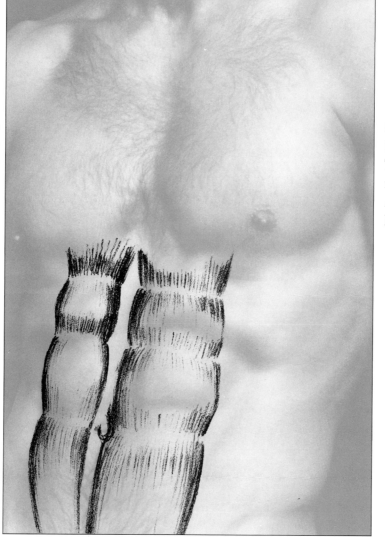

INSERTION: The rectus abdominis inserts at the cartilage of the fifth, sixth, and seventh ribs, and the sternum (xiphoid process).

ORIGIN: The rectus abdominis originates in the crest of the pubis.

MUSCULAR DESCRIPTION: The rectus abdominis runs the length of the AB area, from the pubic bone to the chest.

MOVEMENT: The rectus abdominis pulls the torso toward the hips and the hips toward the torso. It is also responsible for tilting the pelvis, which effects the curvature of the lower back.

EXERCISES: Sit-ups, Crunches, and Reverse Crunches.

PERFORMANCE: Strengthening the rectus abdominis will enhance performance in sports requiring jumping, running, and lifting objects—activities such as Olympic weightlifting, wrestling, pole vault, and high jump.

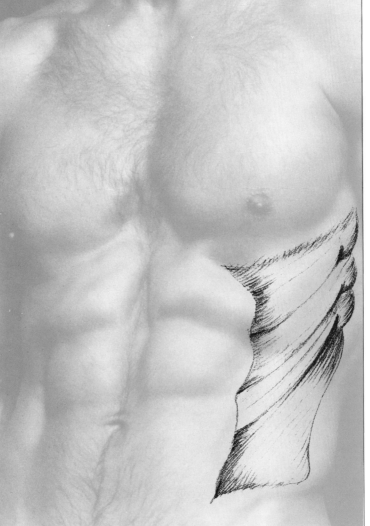

INSERTION: The muscle inserts on the front half of the hip (ilium) and the crest of the pubis. Then it attaches to the tissue of the rectus abdominis.

ORIGIN: The muscle originates from the lower eight ribs and attaches with the serratus muscle that covers the ribs.

MUSCULAR DESCRIPTION: Runs diagonally to the rectus abdominis.

MOVEMENT: The external oblique aids in the twisting of the trunk. The left external oblique is activated when twisting to the right, and the right external oblique is activated when twisting to the left.

EXERCISES: Sit-ups with a Twist, Bicycles, Crossovers.

PERFORMANCE: Strengthening this area will improve performance in such sports as golf, tennis, and baseball, to name a few. It will help you perform any activities where you rotate your trunk.

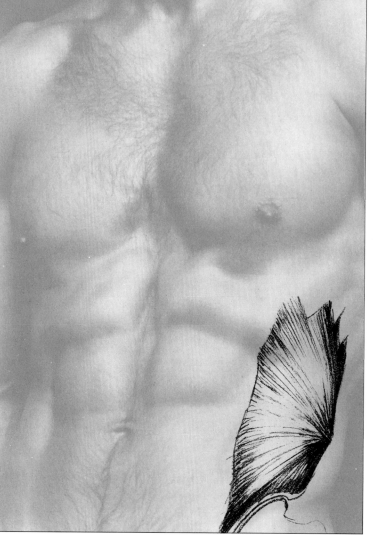

INSERTION: The internal oblique inserts into the cartilages of the eighth, ninth, and tenth ribs.

ORIGIN: The internal oblique originates from top front of the hip (front two thirds of ilium) and the inguinal ligament (which also runs across the front of the hip), connecting with the lumbar tissue.

MUSCULAR DESCRIPTION: The internal oblique lies underneath the external oblique and runs in a diagonally opposed direction.

MOVEMENT: The internal oblique muscles aid the trunk in twisting in the same direction as the side they are on. The left internal oblique helps the torso twist to the left. It aids the right external oblique in this movement. The right internal oblique helps the torso twist to the right, aiding the left external oblique in this movement.

EXERCISES: Hanging Knee Raises with a Cross, Crunches with a Cross, Sit-ups with a Cross.

PERFORMANCE: As with the external oblique, strengthening this muscle will improve your performance in sports where you rotate the trunk, such as skiing, canoeing, soccer.

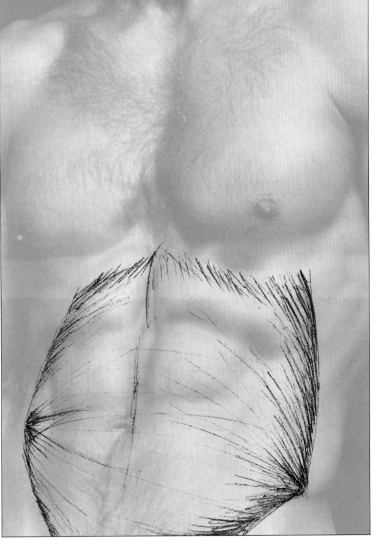

INSERTION: The transverse abdominis inserts on the crest of the pubis.

ORIGIN: The transverse abdominis originates from the rim of the crest of the ilium, the lower six ribs, running along the outer part of the inguinal ligament (which runs across the top of the pelvis), and connects to the lumbar muscle.

MUSCULAR DESCRIPTION: Runs horizontally across the abdominal wall and along the midsection underneath the external and internal obliques.

MOVEMENT: The transverse abdominis pulls the AB wall inward, forcing expiration.

EXERCISES: The vacuum and lower AB movements such as Leg Raises and Knee Raises.

PERFORMANCE: Strengthening the transverse abdominis will enhance performance in sports with short-term power activities such as karate, shot put, and football.

CHAPTER THREE

Proper Training Technique: The Body

by BRETT BRUNGARDT

Proper training technique is essential for a successful workout program. It is important for two key reasons: It provides the best results in the least amount of time, and it decreases the chance of injury during training. This chapter will contain important training principles that are essential for complete AB development.

The Complete ABs Philosophy

To achieve these goals you need to train and condition all the major muscles in your abdomen. Incomplete abdominal training will cause a muscular imbalance or weakness. This can cause bad posture, lower-back pain, and increased chances of injuries.

To achieve proper technique, you must look at the ABs as a system. The muscle groups of the abdominal area are synergistic—they act and react together. In most movements, one muscle group is a prime mover, another group is a secondary mover, and a third may be used as a stabilizer. If you don't work for balanced development, one or more of the muscle groups will not perform optimally.

The Basic Principles

STARTING OUT One of the most frequently asked questions is "Where should I start?" or "Which exercises should I do and how many?" There is no one correct answer. Every person is different. You must experiment to find the correct starting point.

Two principles will help you determine a place to begin.

• When learning a new exercise, use minimal intensity (if possible) and perform it while you are fresh.
• Once that exercise has been mastered *with correct technique,* increase the intensity very gradually, until you can no longer perform the movement for the prescribed number of repetitions or you have a breakdown in technique.

This may sound tedious, but remember: technique is the key to success. Be patient—you will be able to perform more and more exercises with greater ease, and achieve better results when you concentrate on proper technique from the beginning.

Full Range of Motion

It is important to perform all exercises through a full range of motion. You must maintain resistance on the muscles throughout the entire movement. This is especially important for sports performance. Most sports skills are dynamic (in motion), therefore your muscles need to be strengthened throughout their full range of natural motion.

Overload and Progression

Your AB muscles are the same as any other. Training principles don't change. For a muscle to get stronger, it has to be overloaded. Overloading means placing a greater amount of stress on a muscle than it is used to. In simple terms this causes it to adapt and get stronger. Muscle enlargement develops out of necessity. When they are exposed to a greater resistance, they adapt to overcome it. In other words, they get bigger and stronger. Adaptation is synonymous with development. Overloading the AB muscles can be accomplished in two ways, both progressive: First, by either increasing the repetitions per set or adding an exercise to increase total exercise volume; second, by increasing the intensity of training, which can be ac-

complished by increasing the resistance (doing a more difficult exercise or adding weight) or by decreasing the rest time between sets and exercises. These two forms of overloading should be done separately (either increase volume or intensity to create adaptations). When both intensity and volume are increased simultaneously, you are in danger of overtraining.

Speed of Movement

The speed with which you do an exercise is an important part of successful AB training. Generally, the speed should be slow and controlled through both the raising and lowering phases.

As you reach advanced levels of training, it is important to vary the speed of exercise movements to achieve a more complete development. Three basic movement speeds are described in Chapter 9.

Constant Tension

Simply stated, you must maintain constant tension on the muscle, feeling its contraction throughout the full range of motion. Do not let momentum take over. Control the motion, feeling the muscle do the work.

Workout Length

The length of a training session is dependent on total volume, type of exercise, and goals of the individual. You will be provided with a variety of routines to fit your needs and goals. Another variable is intensity. High-intensity work will increase the need for recovery time between exercises, possibly increasing total workout length. Top athletes and bodybuilders generally spend eight to twenty minutes a session specifically training their ABs. Part 4 offers a wide variety of routines from which to choose.

Frequency of Training and Recovery Time Between Workouts

Frequency of training is dependent upon many variables, including recovery time, level of experience, and goals of the exerciser. Recovery time is important because strength gains and muscle growth occur during these periods. If recovery time is not adequate between workouts, strength gains will not be optimal, and over-training can take place. Recovery time is different for each individual, but abdominals can be trained more frequently than most other muscle groups.

Beginners should start by training three times a week. As the exerciser becomes more advanced, you will have to find new ways to increase intensity and volume.

The number of routines can be expanded to five, six, or even seven days of training per week. Just remember that overtraining leads to injuries and burnout. Exercise is for a lifetime, so stay smart and dig in for the long haul. Don't try to do too much too quickly.

Exercise Order

There are many factors to consider when choosing exercise order: sports-specific routines, individual weak areas, fitness levels.

A popular exercise order for ABs is to work lower, oblique, then the upper ABs. Although the ability to completely isolate these groups is questionable, this order makes sense. The exercises are completed in an order of highest energy expenditure to the lowest because you work from the largest muscle areas to the smallest muscle areas.

The Routines

The problem of exercise order, to large extent, is already worked out for you in the routines, but at some point you will want to determine your genetic strengths and weaknesses and choose the exercises for fine-tuning. As with everything else in life, at some point you will be left alone to face the truth about your ABs. But have no fear—you won't fall into the ABs abyss. Chapter 20, "Creating Your Own Routine," will guide you safely through this existential experience!

Warm-up

It is always important to warm your body up before exercising. This prepares your body for action in two ways:

1. *It increases blood flow in the muscle and increases general muscle metabolism. This makes the muscles more efficient.*
2. *It allows the muscles to contract more forcefully and with greater speed due to an increase in muscle temperature. If the muscles are warm, contraction will be optimal. This reduces injury potential.*

For a specific warm-up routine, go to the AB warm-up and stretching routine, page 59.

Breathing

As in all exercising, proper breathing during abdominal training is important. Breathing technique is basically the same as that used when lifting weights. Inhale at the start of the negative contraction, when you are moving against the least resistance; exhale during the last half to two thirds of the positive contraction, when you are moving against the most resistance.

During a crunch, you would exhale as you raise your shoulders off the floor and inhale as you lower your torso.

If this breathing pattern is too difficult, natural breathing during an AB exercise would be satisfactory, but under no circumstances should you hold your breath.

Intensity

Intensity is a complex subject. For our purposes, intensity means the amount of energy it takes to complete an exercise. Intensity can be increased or decreased by choosing easier or more difficult exercises or by adding weight. You should aim for the intensity level that will produce muscular exhaustion in the prescribed number of repetitions, each workout trying to push yourself an extra repetition.

Variation

Variation is often the most neglected training principle. People get comfortable in a routine and don't want to change. We are creatures of habit. But the body thrives on both structure and change. You will start on a routine, and the body will hook into that structure and thrive on it. This will be a growth period. There will be gains in strength, endurance, and/or body appearance. But after a certain period of time, your body will start to adapt to this routine, and stagnate or plateau. This means it's time for a change. The body wants something new. It needs a new routine to challenge and cause adaptation and growth.

Variation also prevents boredom and monotony in training. And hitting the muscles from a variety of angles gives better overall development. Chapter 18, "The Complete Multi-Level System," has variety built into each level.

Repetitions

A repetition is the completion of the entire movement of an exercise. If an athlete performs ten sit-ups, he has completed ten repetitions. Repetitions are also referred to as "reps."

Set

A set is a consecutive series of repetitions. If you perform ten repetitions of the Crunch, rest, and perform another ten repetitions, you have performed two sets of ten repetitions each.

How Much Do I Aim for?

The number of repetitions and sets you do depends on your fitness level and your goals. There is no hard-and-fast rule. Professional bodybuilders and top athletes have gotten results using a wide variety of routines differing in numbers of sets, reps, and exercises. The general consensus for ABs work is to stay between ten and thirty repetitions and between one and five sets per exercise. This allows for a wide variety of groupings and combinations within a routine.

OVERTRAINING Overtraining simply means doing too much and not giving yourself enough rest. It means you have worked the muscle too often and too intensely, not giving it enough time to repair itself. It is

the same as being overworked at the office. You start to become less efficient at your work, and you start to burn out. Sometimes less is more. If you're a certain type of person, it is easy to push yourself too hard, becoming too critical, always wanting more and more. It shouldn't become an unhealthy obsession. Remember, the purpose of exercise is to improve the quality of your life (mentally and physically), not just your appearance. Be patient, train smart, and enjoy every repetition. Get into the process, not just the results.

Quality of the Rep

The most important element in training is not quantity but quality. Don't worry about how many reps you are doing. Concentrate on quality and technique; keep your technique strict, and go through a full range of motion on each repetition. Feel the contraction of each rep; keep constant tension on the AB muscles throughout the movement. Indulge in each and every repetition.

Rest Periods During Workouts

The purpose of rest periods between sets is to recover in order to perform the next set. In general, you should keep your rest time as short as needed for recovery. But again, this depends on your goals and your fitness level. Beginners need more rest time. If you are doing an advanced routine with weight, you will also need more rest time. As a rule of thumb, you should never rest more than sixty seconds between sets. As your fitness level increases, your rest time should decrease from thirty seconds to no rest stops. But remember: Always keep the principle of variety in mind.

Pain

An important part of working out is getting in touch with your body. Part of this experience is learning to distinguish between good pain and bad pain. So be smart and listen to your body.

Good pain is the feeling of being pumped, having the muscle fill with blood. And yes, even that burning sensation that comes from lactic acid buildup. It signals fatigue in the muscle you are working—which is the goal of exercise. These are feelings you will learn to thrive on and may even come to regard as a pleasure.

Bad pain is a warning sign. It means you've injured yourself. When you feel this type of pain, stop immediately. If you have any doubts, its always better to play it safe rather than to risk an injury. If you have lower-back problems, this is something you must be especially careful about. Be aware of your lower back at all times. Warning signs are shooting pains, sharp pains, spasms, and pain that moves into such peripheral areas as legs, arms, feet, or hands. You don't want to push yourself through bad pain. It is a sign that you need to take time off and see a doctor, or change to exercises that don't cause problems.

Soreness

Muscle soreness is common after a workout. Don't worry if you're a little sore (good pain). Soreness is most likely caused by microscopic tears in muscle tissue. They need recuperation time and proper nutrition to repair. The increased blood flow and movement in the area will repair the tissue. If you are too sore to train during your next session, you have overdone it. Train hard, train smart—exercise is for a lifetime.

References

Brungardt, Brett. *The Strength Kit,* 2nd. Edition. Aspen, CO: Strength Advantage, 1990.

O'Bryant, Harold, and Mike Stone. *Weight Training: A Scientific Approach.* Minneapolis: Burgess Publishing Co., 1984.

CHAPTER FOUR

Proper Training Technique: The Mind

by MIKE BRUNGARDT

In any task you undertake, whether it's beginning an exercise program, running a business, or training for a gold medal, the right mental attitude is essential for success. To achieve peak performance, the mind and the body must work together. Ask any champion body-builder, any athlete, any coach. "What is the most important factor in training and performance?" They will all say, "The mind." Mental focus is what separates champions from everybody else.

Planning Your Success

You must have a goal. What you want to look like. How you want to feel. And a time frame in which to accomplish your aspirations. Write these goals down. Remember—*a goal is not a goal unless it is written down.* Then read your goals everyday. It's no use writing them down if you don't read them daily. Read them on days when you're excited about working out, but especially read them on days when you're dragging, when the last thing you want to do is work out. Read them out loud. Own your goals. Take responsibility for them.

You'll find it useful to have long-term, intermediate, short-term goals, and daily tasks:

Long-Term Goals: Write down where you would like to be a year from now. Be specific. For example, one goal might be that you want washboard ABs. You may have a picture from a magazine of how you want to look. Cut it out and paste it next to the written goal.

Intermediate Goals: Write down goals for where you want to be in six months. If you consistently work your ABs for six months, you can accomplish noticeable improvements, so set these goals high.

Short-Term Goals: Write down where you want to be in a month. Every month you need to update this goal, always keeping in mind the end result you want in six months and in a year. Examples of goals you might wish to attain would be losing a certain amount of weight or body fat, achieving a certain degree of firmness and definition, and developing a certain amount of strength and endurance.

Daily Tasks: At the beginning of each day or at night before you go to bed, set at least two goals for the upcoming day. For some, it may be better to plan for the entire week at the beginning of the week. These tasks should be aimed at helping you to achieve your overall goals. Be specific. You should include not only what the task is, but also when it will be performed. For example, on Monday your daily tasks might be: 1) AB workout (specific program) at 6:00 P.M., and 2) Salad and a whole-wheat roll for lunch. This strategy will give you a specific plan designed to help you accomplish your goals.

The Mind-Body Connection

A mind that is programmed for failure will inevitably cause the body to fail. The information you give your subconscious, the images you feed it, will play a big role in determining the result of any endeavor. Great

athletes all know about this connection between their mind and body. Sportscasters describe this state as "playing in a zone." In recent years, sports psychology has developed techniques that help athletes train their minds just as they train their bodies. The techniques that work for them will also help you in your training. The three basic skills are relaxation, concentration or focus, visualization, and power phrases. The techniques will help push you through tough periods.

RELAXATION There are many benefits to be derived from relaxation. It reduces stress and rejuvenates the body. It is also a necessary state for effective visualization. The subconscious is more likely to accept suggestion when you are relaxed. Here are two basic relaxation skills: controlled breathing and progressive relaxation.

CONTROLLED BREATHING One way to achieve a relaxed state is by concentrating on your breathing. Sit or lie down in a comfortable position and focus on inhaling and exhaling for approximately a minute. Then start to inhale on a count of five and exhale on a count of five, until you feel that your breathing pattern is smooth and regular. Then focus on the feeling of air coming into your lungs and imagine it being transported to every cell of your body. Every time you breathe out, let any negative thoughts or feelings you might have leave your body on the breath. Each time you breath in, imagine the breath purifying and energizing your body. If it helps, imagine the breath entering your body as a white cleansing light. Continue this process until you feel a release of muscular tension, a decreased heart rate, rhythmic, calm breathing, and a feeling of being centered. Being centered is a state in which muscular tension is eliminated and the mind is emptied and focused on the moment, allowing you to concentrate solely on the task at hand. Now you are ready for visualization and positive programming.

PROGRESSIVE RELAXATION This technique is a way of consciously programming your body to relax. Lie or sit in a comfortable position, and take a couple of deep breaths. On the exhalations, give your body the message to relax. Then start to feel where your body is making contact with the floor or the chair. If you're lying down, feel your heels, buttocks, shoulders, and head touching the floor. Then move your focus down to your feet. Send the message to the little muscles in the soles of your feet and across the top of your feet to relax. Move up to your calves, and send the message to let your calf muscles relax. Move up to your thighs and hamstrings and tell them to relax. Go to the muscles of your buttocks, telling them to relax. Then move to your lower back, middle back, and upper back, giving your entire back the message to relax. Then send the message to your shoulders, arms, hands, chest, and stomach to relax. And finish with your neck, head, face, and throat. Tell all the little muscles around your eyes, cheeks, and jaws to relax. Tell your forehead and scalp to relax. After you have given your entire body, part by part, the message to relax, allow yourself to go deeper and deeper into relaxation with each breath, giving in to gravity and melting into the floor or chair. If you experience a problem with any particular muscle group, you can use the technique of consciously contracting the tense muscle, then letting it relax. This will help make you aware when the muscle is tense and when it is relaxed.

When you have reached a deep level of relaxation, you are ready for visualization and positive programming. To bring yourself out, say to yourself, "On a count of three, I will open my eyes, feeling relaxed and with a reserve of energy, ready to go on with my day." This technique is good to do with a partner; have him or her speak the words to take you through the process.

VISUALIZATION In a nutshell, visualization is the creation of mental pictures. At an unconscious level, you are constantly creating images. These pictures program and create your self-image. The goal of visualization is to consciously create positive images to help you achieve the goals you want.

To achieve the ABs you want, you must be able to see them in your mind's eye. Your model could be a picture from a magazine, the way you looked a few years ago, someone you saw on the beach, or any combination of these images. What's important is that you create a specific image of the way you want your ABs

to look. It is important to keep an element of truth and realism in your picture. Create an image that fits your genetic type and potential. Create a picture you can believe in with every cell of your body. Your picture can change, evolve, and refine itself.

See everything vividly and in detail. The more vivid the visualization, the more effective it will be. It is essential to use sensory details. Imagine the cuts on your ABs. What do they look like? See the separation of your muscles. See the color of your skin. See the washboard layering of your muscles. Make the snapshot of your ideal ABs as clear as possible.

Imagine how these new ABs make you feel. Feel the tightness in your ABs, the hardness of the muscles. See how others react to them. Walk down the beach with them. See your lover's response.

For this technique to be effective, you must visualize every day (or night), not just when you feel like it. Any negative aspects existing in the subconscious took years to formulate and cannot be released overnight. However, with a consistent visualization strategy, you can begin to change these negative aspects and program for success.

PROGRAMMING POWER PHRASES Power programming is the creation of an affirmation phrase that will help push you to achieve your goals. This phrase doesn't have to be detailed. But it must be evocative enough to eliminate negative thoughts. Phrases such as "I will prevail" or "I am right on track" are examples of power phrases. Avoid using a negative in a power phrase such as, "I will not fail" or "there's no way I'll lose." "No" and "not" are negative programmers, even though the phrase, in its entire context, is positive. Get in the habit of using them extensively, especially when you feel doubts or negative thoughts creeping in your mind. Everyone experiences these doubts. People who succeed fight through their doubts, no matter how extreme they may be. They continue to move forward. Every person has the ability to overcome negative thoughts and doubts, but many people give in to them.

CONCENTRATION OR FOCUS It is amazing how many people can perform an exercise and feel it in an area of the body that is completely unrelated to the movement. When any exercise is performed, if it is performed correctly, the muscles being worked will derive benefits from the movement, regardless of where the mind is focused. But to achieve optimal results, you must concentrate on the area being worked, initiating what is known as the "mind-muscle link." The mind-muscle link is a bridge between your mind and the area you are exercising, which enables your mind and body to work together for a desired result. Metaphorically, it is putting your mind in your muscle. You must focus on the muscles being exercised and feel them in action. You have to be in the moment: Indulge in the sensual side of working out, feel your body move, feel every muscle fiber contract and expand. Get into it, use your imagination, fantasize. Unfortunately, for many people this is easier said than done. In order to initiate this "mind-muscle link," it helps to know where you are placing your focus.

Let's use the crunch movement as an example. As you raise your shoulder blades off the floor, you are causing a contraction primarily in the upper ABs. This is the target area. Your mind should be focused on that area, forming a mind-muscle link. Your mind should not be going over your grocery list. Take one hand and place it on the target area while you perform an exercise. Your hand will transmit the tightening on the concentric contraction to the brain. After a while you will be able to sense this tightening without using your hand to assist. Concentrating on the working body part is one of the most important elements in achieving peak results.

MOTIVATION The mind is the great motivator. The power of the mind will allow you to push through your preconceived limits. This is what will take you to the next level. The techniques discussed in this chapter are designed to help your mind become your strength. A weak mind will talk you out of achieving your goal; a strong mind will guide you to achieve goal after goal after goal. Motivation is very personal. There are tons of tapes, books, and seminars on the subject. And there is also "the well within." Take it where you can get it.

You have to create a vision and work toward it every day, harnessing your unused potential, pushing yourself to places you have never been, step-by-step.

PART TWO

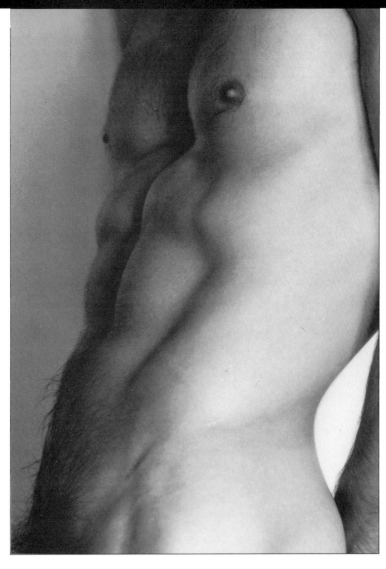

Wellness

MOST NUMBER OF LEG LIFTS IN TWELVE HOURS?

41,785 by Lou Scripa, 1988

CHAPTER FIVE

Complete Nutrition

by BECKY CHASE, M.S., R.D.

Nutrition can make the difference between having enough energy to get by and feeling really good! There are no magical foods or nutritional supplements that will give you a strong, flat abdomen, but eating well will maximize your efforts in the gym. To achieve the abdominal shape you want, *work off what you eat and eat what you work off.* This means working off excess calories and body fat and replacing the essential nutrients used during those workouts

Water—The Single Most Important Nutrient

Sixty percent of an adult's body weight is water. Every metabolic reaction in the body involves water, including the burning of body fat and other fuels for energy.

The body's dependence on water is reflected in the fact that a person can live only three days without it, whereas it is possible to survive many days without food. When a person is low on water—dehydrated— all body functions suffer, including the ability to exercise. Losing as little as 1–2 percent of your body weight through sweat can cause a 10 percent decrease in aerobic capacity—your ability to use oxygen for energy production. As a result, your stamina goes down.

HOW MUCH IS ENOUGH? The average adult uses six to twelve cups of water daily to take care of essential tasks such as removing waste products, transporting nutrients and oxygen throughout the body, and maintaining normal body temperature. This water is lost through urine, breath, sweat, and stools. Exercisers lose even more water, especially if working out in high altitudes or in hot, humid weather. Remember the advertisements for sweat suits in the back of magazines and on late-night TV? "Lose an inch a day while walking your way to slimness in our new exercise-enhancement suits." Well, the term *sweat suit* is appropriate. The heavy suits trapped water, preventing the body from cooling itself through sweat evaporation. The body produced more sweat in an effort to compensate. The inches lost were inches of water! A dehydrated body *appears* slimmer, right up to the moment it passes out from lack of water.

So, be good to yourself and drink plenty of water daily to replace normal fluid losses and to replace the water used during exercise. Most people need eight to ten cups of water daily. This may sound like you will be drowning yourself. Once you get used to drinking plenty of water, you won't mind, because the reward is feeling more energetic.

FLUID OPTIONS While it is important to drink several glasses of plain water each day, you don't have to meet 100 percent of your fluid needs with water. You can use other beverages too—juices, soups, skim milk, herbal tea, decaffeinated coffee, and seltzer water. Even juicy foods help, such as oranges, tomatoes, and cucumbers. Caffeine and alcohol have a diuretic effect on the body, meaning they cause you to make more urine and lose more water. If you drink caffeinated or alcoholic beverages, do so in moderation and do not count them as part of your water intake. How can you be sure you are getting the fluids you need? Your sense of thirst is not always reliable, so monitor your urine output. You should make frequent trips to the bathroom and have clear urine, except for the first void in the morning. You can also follow the guidelines below for water intake during exercise.

Fluid Replacement Guidelines

MODERATE–HEAVY WORKOUTS (1–1½ hours long)

Before: Drink 1–1½ cups of plain cool water 15 minutes before exercise

During: Drink ½ cup of water every 15 minutes

After: Drink 1½–3 cups after exercising, over a 1–2 hour period of time

ENDURANCE EVENTS

Before: Weigh yourself before the event! Drink 3–4 cups of plain cool water during the 2 hours before the event

During: Drink ½ cup of water every 15 minutes Also drink ½ cup of carbohydrate "sports" drink after 1 hour of exercise and every 20–30 minutes

After: Drink 1 cup of water, fruit juice, or "sports" drink every 20 minutes until your pre-event weight is reached or about 2 cups per pound lost

The Energy Nutrients—Your Body's Fuel Source

Energy is measured in food in the form of calories. Fat, carbohydrate, protein, and alcohol all contain calories in varying amounts, as shown in Table 1.

As you can see, fat and alcohol provide more than twice the calories of carbs or protein. Also, current research is telling us that all calories are not created equal. It appears the body is far more efficient in storing fat calories than carbohydrate calories. If you eat one hundred calories of extra fat—say, a tablespoon of margarine—the body stores about ninety-seven of those calories in your fat cells. The other three are lost in the process as heat. (This is called the TEF, or thermal effect of food.) However, if you eat one hundred calories of extra carbs, about two tablespoons of jam, the body stores only seventy-seven calories as fat and loses twenty-three as heat. And, those extra carbs are first stored in muscle and the liver as glycogen. Only when the glycogen stores are full will the carbs be stored as fat. So, fat calories are more fattening than carbohydrate calories. Even if you are not eating any *extra* calories, a low-fat, high-carbohydrate diet allows for a leaner body than a high-fat diet. So, instead of *buttered* toast, eat *jammed* toast.

Burning Fats and Carbs

As you sit and read this book, the calories you are using are slightly more than half fat, and the rest are mostly carbohydrate. Of course, you aren't burning very much of either one, which is why the Read Books and Lose Weight Diet was never a success. Now, if you jump up and sprint to the corner, your body shifts into burning mostly carbs. Should you then decide to walk briskly to the store four miles away, it will start to burn significant amounts of fat along with carbohydrate after about the first mile and a half. If you sprint hard the last quarter-mile, you switch back to using mostly carbs for energy.

Carbohydrate inside the body is in the form of glycogen, stored in muscle and the liver, and glucose (blood sugar). We can store pounds and pounds of fat, but glycogen stores are limited to one pound for the average adult and up to two to three pounds for highly trained athletes. Brain cells rely almost exclusively on glucose for energy. And since carbs are stored in the muscle, they are the most readily available source of energy. So they get used in large amounts during the early stages of exercise, such as in the sprint to the corner. After the body gets *revved up* (the four-mile walk to the store), fat stores begin to break down for energy also. If you continue to increase the intensity of the exercise, another sprint, you would have to use your reserve of carbs (glycogen).

BURNING BODY FAT Fat requires oxygen to be burned, so only aerobic exercises—bicycling, walk-ing, running—will make a dent in body fat. Exercising at light to moderate levels burns a significant percentage of fat, although you never use fat exclusively. You can generally exercise longer if working low to moderately hard, so total calories and total fat expended can be higher than with high-intensity workouts, especially if you are new to the world of exercise.

Weight training and other anaerobic activities, such as fast sprints, also work to improve the body's lean-to-fat ratio. Weight training, including your abdominal routine, builds muscle. Muscle tissues burn more calories than fat tissues. The more muscle you have, the more calories you will burn, even while sitting. And since nearly half of those calories are fat, you will burn more total fat. High-intensity workouts improve your ability to utilize oxygen during intense exercise, again increasing the use of fat as a fuel.

Protein Builds Muscle, Right?

You've seen the advertisements. An extremely well-developed man with perfect *cut* is touting protein powder as the reason for his incredible physique. Everyone knows muscle is made of protein, so it is logical to assume you need to eat more protein if you want to build muscle. And that is true, but not to the extent many people believe.

Exercisers require more of protein than nonexercisers, with endurance athletes and bodybuilders requiring the most. Sedentary adults need 0.4 gram of protein per pound of body weight and exercisers

TABLE 1. WHERE CALORIES COME FROM			
	CALORIES/GRAM	CALORIES/TBSP.	SOME FOOD SOURCES
FAT	9	120 (oil)	Oil, butter, mayo, cream, bacon, fatty meat, and margarine
CARBOHYDRATE	4	46 (sugar)	Grains, vegetables, fruits, legumes (beans and peas)
PROTEIN	4	*	Meats, milk, cheese, legumes, nuts, grains
ALCOHOL	7	*	Wine, beer, whiskey

*Tablespoon measurements do not apply to protein and alcohol.

Figure 1. Fuels Burned During Exercise

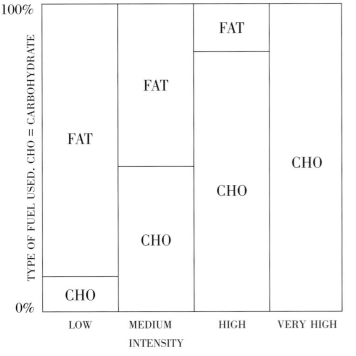

require 0.6 to 0.9 gram per pound. If you are a 150-pound bodybuilder, your maximum protein requirement is 135 grams. I often see men who eat that much protein without even trying! Virtually all foods, except fruit, pure sugars, and pure fats, contain some protein. Table 2 gives the protein content of some common foods.

Although protein has the potential to supply energy, the body has to spare protein for its more important functions, such as the building and repair of tissue and the formation of enzymes, hormones, and other important compounds. At rest, the body uses protein for only 2–5 percent of its calories. Endurance activities will increase protein's usage because protein can be converted into glucose. If an athlete fails to eat adequate carbohydrate, his or her usage of protein for energy will increase. This takes protein away from its other duties and can lead to dehydration and calcium losses. Excess protein can also be stored as body fat. So, eat *enough* protein, but not too much. Generally, protein intake is safe and adequate if no more than 10–20 percent of total calories.

What About Alcohol?

Alcohol is a concentrated source of calories and has negative consequences when consumed in excess. When alcohol enters the body, it acts like an obnoxious jerk, insisting that the liver take care of it while other work comes to a standstill. As a result, fat metabolism slows down, leading to a buildup of fat in the liver. Also, alcohol metabolism ties up niacin and thiamin, B vitamins necessary for energy production. This can make it difficult to exercise after a night of drinking. Also, muscle cells do not use alcohol for energy, so you cannot burn off a martini in the same way you can burn off a doughnut. Instead, the martini is converted to fatty acids. And remember, alcohol has a *diuretic* effect on the body.

Small amounts of alcohol, up to two drinks, may help you feel calm and better able to handle the world. Larger amounts can wreak havoc. If you are going to drink, don't do it right before or after exercise. When participating in a beer-sponsored sporting event, be sure to rehydrate your body with plenty of water before hitting the free beer!

Choosing Foods to Maximize Energy and Minimize Body Fat

You now know where calories come from, but what is the best way to balance them for maximum energy lev-

TABLE 2. PROTEIN CONTENT OF SELECTED FOODS	
FOOD	PROTEIN (grams)
Canned tuna, 6.5 oz. can	45.5
Chicken breast, 4 oz.	36.0
Refried beans, 1 cup	15.8
Broccoli, cooked, 1 cup	5.8
Brown rice, 1 cup	4.9
Whole-wheat bread, 2 slices	4.8
Green beans, 1 cup	2.4
Baked potato, 1 medium	2.0

els? The body uses up more grams of carbohydrate than any other fuel. Since our storage volume of glycogen is limited, we need to replace the glycogen used during exercise as well as provide plenty of glucose to maintain blood-sugar levels. The only way to replace carbs is to eat carbs. We don't need to worry about replacing the fat we burned; we will always have plenty of fat on board.

CARBOHYDRATES There are two kinds of carbohydrates in food—simple and complex. Simple carbs are sugars and fruit. They are simple in their chemical structure, just two molecules hooked together—O-O. Simple carbs are digested and absorbed into the bloodstream very quickly, which is why people talk about getting an *energy high* from sugary foods. The blood sugar rises very quickly, giving the body quick energy. One downside to simple carbs is that some people also get a corresponding *energy low* (from a drop in blood sugar) if they eat too many simple carbs or eat them without other foods.

Complex carbs consist of long strings of molecules, and therefore take longer to digest and absorb. Consequently, the rise in blood sugar is lower and slower, providing a longer-lasting energy. Complex carbs are found in foods such as breads, noodles, cereals, potatoes, corn, beans, and peas. At least 60 percent of an exerciser's calories should be carbohydrate calories, with the majority of those being complex carbs. Plenty of grains, vegetables, and legumes should fill your plate. Fruits are important too, because even though they are mostly simple carbs, they provide necessary fiber, vitamins, and minerals.

SUGARS Sugars are basically devoid of any nutritional value other than simple carbs, making them *empty calories.* Too many empty calories spell DEATH to a well-balanced diet. A little sugar is okay if you are active enough to afford the extra calories—say, one or two servings of sugary junk food a day. More than that will compromise nutrient intake.

FATS—A LITTLE DAB WILL DO YA! Now that you are working hard to have a lean body, the last thing you want to do is refeed your fat cells. Any extra calories can become stored fat, but remember that fat calories get stored most readily. Many people have the mistaken idea that they should not eat *any* fat. This is simply not true! Fat is a necessary part of a well-balanced diet, but a little goes a long way.

Body Fat: Fat has such a bad reputation these days, perhaps it would be helpful for you to understand why fat is important for good health. A certain amount of body fat is essential to life. Body fat protects internal organs, helps to maintain body temperature, and is a vital component of all body cells.

Although estimates vary, men probably require a minimum of 5 percent fat weight, and women require 8 percent body fat to sustain life. Optimal fitness is likely achieved with body-fat levels higher than the minimum, 10–25 percent for men and 15–30 percent for women. These are pretty liberal ranges compared to what some experts recommend. However, people vary greatly in how healthy they are at certain body weights and body fats. We tend to forget this fact in our fat-phobic society. I have known exercisers who feel too lethargic and get sick more often when their body fat gets lower than optimum for them. As you work to achieve the look you want, pay attention to how your body feels. You may be more comfortable at a slightly higher body fat than shooting for the lowest level you can achieve.

So, How Much Fat and What Kind of Fat Should You Eat? We need some food fat to supply essential fat-soluble vitamins and fatty acids required to make hormones and other compounds necessary for life and optimal health. Technically, a healthy diet could be as low as 5 percent fat calories. Practically speaking, a diet that low in fat would have problems. Food fat helps you feel satisfied after eating, and because it slows down digestion, fat keeps you from being hungry all the time. Fat also contributes a lot of flavor. It is widely distributed in foods. You will find some fat in nearly all foods except pure sugars—honey, table sugar, molasses, etc. So every piece of whole-grain bread and every ounce of lean tuna will provide some fat. In order for an exerciser to get the calories he needs with a wide variety of tasty foods, fat intake

TABLE 3. HOW MUCH FAT CAN I EAT?

First, estimate your total calorie needs and the number of fat calories. Then figure grams of fat to eat daily. It is best to calculate a range of intakes instead of a single number.

1. Multiply your weight by the appropriate factor to estimate baseline calorie needs.

Men: 11 _____ lb x 11 = _____

Women: 10 _____ lb x 10 = _____

2. Multiply your weight by the appropriate *activity factor* to estimate calories needed for activity.

	Sedentary	Light	Moderate	Heavy
Men:	3.2	6	7.2	10.5
Women:	3.0	5	6	9

_____ lb x _____ (factor) = _____

3. Add together the calories from 1 and 2 to estimate *total calorie needs* per day.

_____ + _____ = _____

4. Multiply the total calories by .10, .20, or .30 for 10 percent, 20 percent, or 30 percent fat calories.*

_____ x .10 = _____

_____ x .20 = _____

_____ x .30 = _____

5. Divide the calories from fat by 9 to get the number of fat grams to eat per day.

10 percent = _____ /9 = _____

20 percent = _____ /9 = _____

30 percent = _____ /9 = _____

*Eat between 10 percent and 20 percent fat calories to help lose excess body fat.

EXAMPLE

135-lb moderately active female

135 lb x 10 = 1,350 Baseline Calories

135 lb x 6 = 810 Activity Calories

1,350 + 810 = 2,160 Total Calories

2,160 x .10 = 216 Fat Calories (10 percent)

2,160 x .20 = 432 Fat Calories (20 percent)

2,160 x .30 = 648 Fat Calories (30 percent)

216/9 = 24 Fat Grams for 10 percent

432/9 = 48 Fat Grams for 20 percent

648/9 = 72 Fat Grams for 30 percent

probably needs to be at least 10 percent of calories. For good health and disease prevention, limit fat intake to no more than 30 percent of calories. If you need to lose body fat, shoot for 10-20 percent fat calories.

Figuring Your Recommended Fat Intake: Once you decide what percentage of fat calories to eat, it is useful to translate that information into *grams* of fat. Food labels and calorie charts list grams of fat in foods, so you can count your fat intake easily. Table 3 provides a quick method for estimating how many grams of fat you can eat and still be within the percentage of fat calories you want.

Types of Food Fat: After learning the amount of fat to eat, your next consideration is the *type* of fat. Three types of fatty acids give us calories—saturated (SAT), polyunsaturated (POLY), and monounsaturated (MONO). The difference between the three chemically has to do with the amount of hydrogen ions attached. If a fat has all the hydrogens it can handle, it is considered *saturated*. If only one hydrogen is missing, it is a *monounsaturated* fat, and if several hydrogens are missing, it is *polyunsaturated*.

Health Issues: The significance healthwise is that SATs tend to increase blood cholesterol, especially LDL-cholesterol—the harmful kind. SATs are found predominantly in fatty animal products, such as cheese, whole milk, and fatty meats. The recent good news about fat is that the predominant saturated fatty acid in beef and chocolate, stearic acid, does not seem to affect LDL-cholesterol. So feel free to enjoy lean beef and the occasional chocolate bar. POLYs are the type of fat in most plants, except coconut and palm oil, which are saturated. When saturated fats in the diet are replaced with polyunsaturated ones, LDL-cholesterol declines. The same is true if MONOs replace SATs. Olive oil and canola oil are two predominant sources of MONOs.

You have probably seen the term *hydrogenated* on labels of shortening, margarine, and other foods. *Hydrogenated* is the term used when man *saturates* a plant oil by adding hydrogens. Controversy exists about the health effects of hydrogenated fats. It is probably a good idea to use oil instead of shortening when possible, but the most important point is to not use very much of either.

This fatty-acid stuff can get pretty technical. The important thing for you to know is that too much of any fat is too much. The fats that you do eat should be about half MONOs and one fourth each from POLYs and SATs. This means use small amounts of olive or canola oil in cooking and salad dressings, eat only lean animal products, and the PUFAs will take care of themselves through the fat found in grains and vegetables and processed foods.

Cholesterol: Cholesterol is another type of fat that affects heart health but does not provide calories. Many experts consider total fat in the diet more important than total cholesterol, but limiting cholesterol intake to 300 mg per day is still recommended. This is especially important if you already have a high blood-cholesterol level or if it runs in your immediate family. Cholesterol is made in the liver of animals, including humans. Since plants do not have livers, food cholesterol is found only in animal products. It is possible for a food to be high in fat and low in cholesterol—oil, for example. It is also possible to have a high-cholesterol, low-fat food—boiled shrimp. Shrimp, calamari

TABLE 4. PRIMARY SOURCES OF FOOD FAT		
SATURATED	MONO-UNSATURATED	POLY-UNSATURATED
Butter	Olives	Safflower Oil
Cream	Olive Oil	Sunflower Oil
Coconut Oil	Canola Oil	Corn Oil
Palm Oil		Soybean Oil
Whole Milk		Peanut Oil
Cheese		Fish Oil
Bacon, Sausage		Walnuts
Poultry Skin		
Lard		
Beef		
Pork		
Lamb		

(squid), organ meats, and egg yolks are some of the biggest contributors of cholesterol in our diet, so go easy on them.

PROTEIN—MEAT-EATERS VERSUS VEGE-TARIANS The debate is lively and often heated. Should humans eat meat or not? Research indicates many of the life-threatening diseases in the United States could be diminished if we ate fewer animal products, both animal fats and animal proteins. The key word here is *fewer,* not *none.* Since the Stone Age, humans have been omnivorous, able to digest and absorb nutrients from animals as well as plants. (Of course, there were no processed foods then, so diets were lower in fat, sugar, and salt.) A healthy diet can be achieved with or without animal flesh or animal milk. The key is knowing how to choose a nutrient-rich diet.

Body protein is made by putting together various amino acids according to specific directions. Your body is programmed to do this, assuming all the necessary amino acids are available. Most amino acids can be produced by the body, but there are several that have to be supplied from food, the so-called *essential amino acids.* The advantage of animal protein is that it contains all of them, being *a complete protein.* Plants only have some of the essential amino acids and are known as *incomplete proteins.* But you do not have to eat a complete protein in order for your body to make the proteins it needs. After you eat a steak, for example, the process of digestion breaks apart the complete protein, and you absorb individual amino acids and pairs of amino acids. These enter the body's pool of amino acids. When you need a protein built, the body will draw the necessary amino acids from this pool. As long as you obtain all the essential amino acids in enough quantity over the course of the day, it doesn't matter if they originally came from an animal or a plant.

Combining Proteins: Recent research indicates that it is not necessary to combine certain plants at each meal to equal the amino acid content of a complete protein. However, it is very easy to do. Any combination of grains and legumes, legumes and seeds, or dairy protein and plant protein make a complete pro-

tein. The following are examples of complete protein dishes common to the vegetarian diet:

TABLE 5. COMPLETE VEGETARIAN PROTEINS	
Black Beans and Rice	Rice Pudding
Peanut Butter Sandwich	Noodles with Tofu Sauce
Bean Taco	Lentil Curry on Rice
Hummus on Pita Bread	Cereal and Milk
Macaroni and Cheese	Noodles with Peanut Sauce

Pros and Cons of Plant and Animal Proteins: Plant proteins, except for nuts and seeds, are usually very low in fat. However, today many red meats are also quite lean, as are certain fish, skinless poultry, and nonfat dairy products. Vegetarians are not guaranteed a low-fat diet; they have to select foods as carefully as meat-eaters do.

An advantage to plant foods high in protein is that most of them are also high in complex carbohydrates. It is like eating meat and bread all at once when you choose to eat a bowl of beans, for example. Of course, you have to eat two cups of beans to get the same amount of protein found in four ounces of chicken. So you may have to consume a greater volume of food to meet your protein needs with a vegetarian diet. On the other hand, vegetarians are less likely to overdo it on protein unless large amounts of eggs, milk, and cheese are consumed. Arguments can be made in favor of both vegetarian and meat diets. The important thing is to eat adequate but not excessive protein.

Putting It All Together— A Well-Balanced Diet

So what exactly is a well-balanced diet? There is so much conflicting information about nutrition, it can be difficult to get a clear grasp on they answer to that question. As more is learned about our nutritional needs in fighting disease, the message of exactly what to eat gets confusing for consumers. Well, you know the old adage—*Keep it simple, Sherlock.* It is applicable in nutrition, as in most things. The majority of the population could vastly improve their nutritional status by simply getting back to the basics—i.e., eating a variety of whole, unprocessed foods. This requires eating baked potatoes instead of potato chips.

There are at least forty nutrients essential to life. Other compounds, not yet considered nutrients, are being investigated for their role in promoting optimal health. No single food or limited group of foods offers all these nutrients and compounds, making variety a very important part of good nutrition.

GET THE BIGGEST NUTRITIONAL BANG FOR YOUR BUCK We require fewer calories than our ancestors because we are less physical. However, our need for vitamins, minerals, and fiber has not decreased. This creates a situation where we need to get as many nutrients per calorie as possible, a principle known as *nutrient density*. But as our need for calories has decreased, our foods have become more processed. Processed foods typically provide fewer nutrients per calorie than whole foods. See Table 6 for examples. Eating foods that are close to their original form is the best way to increase nutrient density.

Surveys vary in their estimate of the percentage of the American population that eats a well-balanced diet, but by all accounts it is well below 50 percent. Some people complain that eating well is too complicated, and others say healthy foods don't taste good. As for the how-to part, follow this rule: *Choose more of the best and less of the rest,* meaning choose mostly wholesome, *real* foods, and eat the processed junk food less often. Instead of instant macaroni and cheese, eat noodles topped with chicken and veggies. Have pudding made with skim or low-fat milk for dessert instead of creme-filled sandwich cookies.

As for good taste, you may have to reacquaint your taste buds with the flavor of real food. But what could taste better than a juicy peach, fresh steamed asparagus, a salad of mixed greens, or a bowl of pasta with spaghetti sauce? The spaghetti sauce can even contain meatballs and still be lean, healthy, and delicious. Use the Power Nutrition guidelines on the next page to achieve a diet full of vital nutrients without a lot of unnecessary calories. The sample menus demonstrate how to create meals that add up to that elusive *well-balanced diet.*

BALANCED CALORIES EQUAL BETTER ENERGY You will notice that in each of the sample menus, the meals contain plenty of carbohydrates along with some protein. I have found that most people feel more energetic when they eat a mixed meal instead of just carbs or mostly protein. Mixed meals offer a longer-lasting supply of blood sugar. A currently popular approach to nutrition is to *not* combine starches and meats, and to eat only fruit in the mornings. A few of my clients swear by this approach, but the majority do not, especially if they are exercising hard. Blood-sugar lows can occur when eating just fruit, and the menu limitations with this approach are unnecessary. The bottom line is to get all the nutrients you need and to feel good. *To combine or not to combine is a personal choice.*

TABLE 6. COMPARISON OF SELECTED NUTRIENTS PER 100 CALORIES					
	FAT (GM)	POTASSIUM (MG)	ZINC (MG)	IRON (MG)	VITAMIN B6 (MG)
Baked Potato	0.1	384	0.29	1.25	0.32
French Fries	5.2	232	0.12	0.24	0.07
Potato Chips	6.8	249	0.20	0.22	0.09
Corn on the Cob	0.8	315	0.70	0.70	0.18
Creamed Corn	0.5	185	0.70	0.50	0.09
Whole-Wheat Bread	1.8	72	0.69	1.4	0.08
White Bread	1.4	42	0.23	1.1	0.00

Data adapted from *Food Values of Portions Commonly Used,* 15th edition.

PLANNING TIPS Healthy meals don't just happen unless you think *nutrition* when you think about food. Planning menus ahead is an invaluable tool in helping you stay on track with a healthy eating plan. You may shy away from planning because of the time involved, but I spend less than one hour a week planning menus. That hour saves me time later in trying to figure out what to cook. Also, if I am tired at the end of the day and haven't preplanned dinner, I am more likely to opt for a quick dinner out or a frozen pizza. However, if I have decided ahead what to cook, it is pretty easy to get a healthy dinner on the table. Here are some simple strategies for planning and preparing healthy menus:

POWER NUTRITION MEANS CHOOSING MORE OF THE BEST AND LESS OF THE REST
(Part 1)

ANIMAL PROTEIN		PLANT PROTEIN		DAIRY PROTEIN	
3–6 oz. Total per Day	Serving Size	Use 2–3 Times per Week in Place of Animal Protein	Serving Sizes Are Equal in Protein to 1 Ounce of Meat	2–4 Servings per Day (high in calcium)	Serving Size Is Equal in Protein to 1 Ounce of Meat
0–1 GRAM OF FAT*		0–1 GRAM OF FAT*		0–1 GRAM OF FAT*	
Egg white	1 egg white	**Legumes, beans and	¹/₂ cup	Milk, nonfat powder	¹/₄ cup
Flounder or sole, baked	3 ounces	peas, dried or canned		Milk, skim	1 cup
Oysters, raw	3 ounces	and cooked without		Yogurt, plain, nonfat	1 cup
Shrimp, boiled	3 ounces	added fat		Evaporated skimmed milk	¹/₂ cup
				Fat-free cheeses	1–1¹/₂ ounces
				Fat-free cream cheese	2 ounces
3–5 GRAMS OF FAT*		3–5 GRAMS OF FAT*		3 GRAMS OF FAT*	
Skinless chicken or turkey,	3 ounces	**Miso, fermented	3¹/₂ ounces	Milk, 1 percent	1 cup
baked or roasted		**Tempeh	1¹/₂ ounces	Cottage cheese	¹/₄ cup
Most fish and shellfish, boiled	3 ounces	**Tofu	3¹/₂ ounces	Yogurt, fruit-flavored,	1 cup
or cooked without fat				low-fat	
Canned tuna or salmon	3 ounces				
(**with bones)					
Egg, whole	1 egg				
Lean beef, lean pork, ham	3 ounces				
8–10 GRAMS OF FAT*		15–20 GRAMS OF FAT*		5 GRAMS OF FAT*	
Chicken, fried	3 ounces	Nuts	1 ounce (¹/₄–¹/₃ cup)	Cheese, skim mozzarella	1 ounce
Kippered herring	3 ounces	Peanut butter	2 Tbsp.	Cheese, reduced	1 ounce
Mackerel, canned	3 ounces	Seeds	1 ounce (¹/₄ cup)	fat varieties	
Oysters, fried	3 ounces			Milk, 2 percent	1 cup
Sardines**	3 ounces			Yogurt, plain, low-fat	1 cup
Salmon, baked	3 ounces				
Shrimp, fried	3 ounces				
Steak, broiled	3 ounces				
15–20 GRAMS OF FAT*				10 GRAMS OF FAT*	
Beef, ground and roasts with	3 ounces			Cheese, regular	1 ounce
fat untrimmed.				Milk, whole	1 cup
Hot dogs	2–3 ounces			Yogurt, whole, plain	1 cup
Luncheon meats	2–3 ounces			Milkshake	¹/₄ cup
Sausages	2–3 ounces				

*These are average grams of fat for food within each category.

**Nondairy foods high in calcium. If you do not consume dairy products, it is important to get several other good sources of calcium every day.

- Look through cookbooks to select recipes/dishes. Select four or five dinner meals for the week.
- Shop according to the recipes so that you have everything you need on hand.
- Prepare extra amounts of foods that are called for in more than one dish. For example, you could have baked chicken with rice and then use the leftovers to make a vegetable/chicken stir-fry.
- Always cook enough for leftovers. Use these for the next day's lunch whenever possible. Freeze the rest for an easy meal later. You can even make your own TV dinners by freezing individual meals on divided plates.
- At lunchtime, ask yourself what you ate for breakfast and what you plan to eat for dinner. Use lunch to make up for any missing food groups.
- Keep plenty of quick breakfast and lunch items on hand to fill in when there are no leftovers. Some suggestions are listed below.

SURVIVING THE GROCERY STORE

I actually *enjoy* going to the grocery store, checking out the new products, and selecting healthy, delicious foods. Most people view grocery shopping as a tedious chore that they try to get through as quickly as possible. They buy the same foods over and over only to find themselves bored with the task of putting food on the table. It doesn't have to be that way!

The next time you go grocery shopping:

- Go when you are not already exhausted.
- Always have a shopping list to ease the trauma of decision-making.
- Allow yourself plenty of time. Read a few food labels and get acquainted with new products. Comparison-shop on the basis of fat grams and ingredients in addition to price. For example, if you are looking for a granola bar, choose one that lists a real food as the first ingredient—fruit or whole grain—as opposed to a sugar. Then check the fat grams before deciding which brand to buy.
- Plan to purchase one new food—a new vegetable or low-fat item. The natural foods aisle is a great place to explore. You will find unusual grains, as well as some healthy convenience foods.

QUICK BREAKFAST FOODS TO KEEP ON HAND

A variety of dry cereals	Fresh fruit
Skim milk	Frozen juices
Nonfat or low-fat yogurt	Eggs or frozen egg substitute
Frozen, unsweetened fruit	Pancake mix and lower-sugar
Bagels	syrup
Fat-free cream cheese	Raisins and other dried fruits
Granola bars	Whole-grain bread

- Leave the kids at home! Think of it as a minivacation, some time alone.
- Don't go with a ravenous appetite or an overly full belly. If you arrive at the store hungry, take the time to get a snack before you start shopping.

THINGS TO CONSIDER ON A FOOD LABEL

The food-labeling laws are currently in revision, and you should see the improved version by mid-1993. Here are some basics to know:

- Ingredients are listed in descending order by weight. The item listed first is present in the largest amount, based on weight, not volume or calories.
- The bold print is marketing. Even though health claims are regulated by law, food companies take as much liberty as possible in promoting their products. Read the nutritional information before deciding if the product meets your standards.
- Pay attention to serving size. Did you know a can of soda is usually considered two servings? Who drinks half a can of pop? Currently, serving sizes are not

---

QUICK LUNCH FOODS TO KEEP ON HAND

Instant soups—Nile Spice or Fantastic Foods Brands

Tabbouleh salad mix (use half the oil)

Pocket bread (fill with tabbouleh or veggies)

Fresh veggies—tomatoes, onions, cucumbers, lettuce, carrots

Canned beans or low-fat refried beans

Tortillas (for bean burritos)

Nonfat or low-fat cheese

Whole-grain crackers

Peanut butter, the natural kind

Low-fat frozen meals by Healthy Choice, Lean Cuisine, Le Menu Light, etc.

SAMPLE MENUS*

MENU 1 12% Fat Calories	MENU 2 23% Fat Calories	MENU 3 Vegetarian (23% Fat)
MEAL 1: ¹/₂ cup orange juice 1 cup oatmeal with 1 Tbsp. raisins and 1 Tbsp. blackstrap molasses 2 slices whole-wheat toast with 1 Tbsp. jam 1 cup skim milk	MEAL 1: ¹/₂ cup orange juice 1 cup oatmeal with 1 Tbsp. raisins, 1 Tbsp. molasses **and ¹/₂ Tbsp. margarine** 2 slices whole-wheat toast with 1 Tbsp. jam 1 cup skim milk	MEAL 1: ¹/₂ cup orange juice 1 cup oatmeal with 1 Tbsp. raisins, 1 Tbsp. molasses and ¹/₂ Tbsp. margarine 2 slices whole-wheat toast with 1 Tbsp. jam 1 cup skim milk
MEAL 2: Tuna-fish sandwich with: 2 ounces tuna, 2 slices whole-wheat bread, 1 Tbsp. low-fat mayonnaise, lots of lettuce and tomato slices 1 raw carrot	MEAL 2: Tuna-fish sandwich with: 2 ounces tuna, 2 slices whole-wheat bread, **1 Tbsp. regular mayonnaise,** lots of lettuce and tomato slices 1 raw carrot 1 ounce pretzels 1 cup lemonade	MEAL 2: **2 bean burritos made with 1 cup black beans, 2 flour tortillas, lettuce, tomato, and avocado** 1 cup lemonade
SNACK 1: 1 banana sliced into 1 cup nonfat yogurt with 1 tsp. honey	SNACK 1: 1 banana sliced into 1 cup nonfat yogurt with 1 tsp. honey	SNACK 1: 1 banana sliced into 1 cup nonfat yogurt with 1 tsp. honey
MEAL 3: 1¹/₂ cups noodles topped with 2 ounces cooked chicken breast, 1¹/₈ cups mixed vegetables cooked in 1 tsp. olive oil 1 slice French bread topped with 1 clove baked garlic 4 ounces white wine	MEAL 3: **1 cup noodles** topped with 2 ounces chicken breast, 1¹/₈ cups mixed vegetables cooked in 1 tsp. olive oil, and **1 Tbsp. Parmesan cheese** **Water**	MEAL 3: 1 cup noodles topped with **2 ounces tofu,** 1¹/₈ cups mixed vegetables cooked in 1 tsp. olive oil, and 1 Tbsp. Parmesan cheese 1 slice French bread with 1 tsp. margarine Water
SNACK 2: 1 apple 1 cup herbal tea	SNACK 2: 1 apple 1 cup herbal tea	SNACK 2: 1 apple 1 cup herbal tea
2,094 calories 12% fat calories 67% carb calories 18% protein calories 3% alcohol calories	2,107 calories 23% fat calories 60% carbohydrate calories 17% protein calories 0% alcohol calories	2,142 calories 20% fat calories 65% carbohydrate calories 15% protein calories 0% alcohol calories

*Note that as fat is added, carbohydrate, protein, and alcohol must decrease to compensate. Each menu meets the Power Nutrition guidelines. Bold print indicates how the menu differs from previous menu.

standardized for all foods, although this will change under the new rules. In the meantime, some products list a smaller serving size so that calories and fat appear lower.

- A product contains less than 30 percent calories from fat if it has only three grams of fat per hundred calories. Not every food you eat has to be low-fat, but it is helpful to compare fat grams, especially in convenience-type products.
- When the bold print says *93 percent fat free, 7 percent fat,* it is usually referring to fat by weight, not by calories. You will often see this on meat products. The fat by calories could be way over 30 percent. Check the fat and calories per serving to decide if it is a low-fat product.
- Be aware that many low-fat products have traded sugar and additives for the fat. Just because a food is low-fat doesn't make it healthy. Low-fat junk food is still junk food. Use it only occasionally.

When to Eat What—Timing Your Meal with Exercise

What you eat and when you eat it in relation to your workouts can make a big difference in how an exercise session goes. When exercising, your body shifts blood flow away from the digestive tract to the working muscles. Food digestion takes a backseat, and you will want to time your meals accordingly.

FOOD BEFORE EXERCISE Most of the energy used during a workout comes from your stores of glycogen and fat. However, if you exercise longer than one hour, a pre-exercise meal can contribute necessary glucose for long workouts. Some research indicates that overweight people benefit more from exercise if they eat after exercise, not before. The exercise tends to increase the TEF of the following meal, causing you to waste more of those calories as heat. Exercise may also help control appetite for the following meal. On the other hand, if you decide to take a run first thing in the morning, you will be low on glycogen stores from your overnight fast. A light, high-carbohydrate meal, perhaps a bagel with jam one hour before, will help abate hunger and prevent low blood sugar. If exercising at low-to-moderate intensity, you will probably feel fine on an empty stomach, provided you ate a high-carbohydrate meal the night before.

If you do eat before exercise, make it a low-fat meal to enhance digestion. Fiber is another consideration. A high-fiber meal may lead to bloating and discomfort if eaten too close to the exercise session. You will have to experiment with what works best for you. A rule of thumb to follow for pre-exercise meals:

- If eating less than one hour before, choose a light snack, such as half a bagel or one slice of toast with jam.
- If eating one to two hours before, choose a liquid meal, such as a fruit and milk shake. Liquids leave the stomach sooner than solid.
- If eating two to three hours before, choose a small meal, such as cereal with fruit and milk, toast, and juice.
- If eating three to four hours before, choose a larger meal, such as a turkey sandwich, tossed salad, pretzels, and milk.

Remember to always eat a high-carbohydrate diet to maintain glycogen stores.

What About Sugar and Exercise? If you down a large glass of juice or soda before exercising, you may experience a corresponding low blood sugar, which can lead to dizziness and nausea. This can be quite uncomfortable and interfere with a workout. People vary in their sensitivity to sugar pre-exercise, but it is generally considered a good idea to avoid it. If you want something sweet, have it either two hours before or only a few minutes before your workout, to avoid a sudden drop in blood sugar.

Endurance training, exercise lasting longer than one-and-a-half hours, may be enhanced by drinking low sugar sports drinks for some of your water during the training session. The small amounts of sugar help prolong exercise by providing a ready source of energy to the muscles and maintaining blood-sugar levels. Sports drinks vary in the source of carbohydrate: glucose, glucose polymers, fructose, maltodextrins, or sucrose. How much better is one source over another? That question is still being debated. The important thing is to use these drinks if they are helpful and if you really need them; otherwise, they contribute unnecessary calories with the water you need. Glucose polymers (Exceed brand) may cause less stomach discomfort than fructose-based beverages (ReHydrate brand). However, individual tolerance is the critical factor in choosing a sports drink.

EATING AFTER EXERCISE This is the time to feed your muscle cells, and they like carbs! The first two hours after heavy exercise is the best time to replenish glycogen stores. The muscle cells are ravenous, as well as thirsty, if you have worked long and hard. The first meal following exercise should be primarily carbohydrate—bean soup, rolls, and fruit, for example, instead of a cheeseburger and fries. Also, if you want a soda, this is the time to have it. All that sugar will be gobbled up by your muscle cells. Drink-

POWER NUTRITION MEANS CHOOSING MORE OF THE BEST AND LESS OF THE REST
(Part 2)

CEREALS/GRAINS/BREADS/CRACKERS	
6–11 Servings per Day	
0–2 GRAMS OF FAT*	Serving Size
Whole-grain, low-sugar cereals, such as Bran Flakes, Grape Nuts; Cornflakes, Cheerios, Shredded Wheat, etc.	1 ounce (1/3 to 1 cup usually)
Whole-grain cooked cereals: oatmeal, grits, Cream of Wheat, etc.	1/2 cup cooked
Whole-grain or enriched breads without added cheese or egg.	1 slice (1 ounce)
Whole-grain or enriched noodles, rice, millet, quinoa, etc.	1/2 cup cooked
Bagels, pita bread, corn tortillas	1 each
English muffins, hard rolls, hamburger/hot-dog buns.	1/2 each
Saltine crackers	4 crackers
Whole-grain crackers, no added fat	2–4 crackers
3–5 GRAMS OF FAT*	Serving Size
Biscuit	1 biscuit
Croutons	1/2–1 ounce
Dinner roll	1 roll
Pancakes	4-inch pancake
Granola	1 ounce
Granola bar	1 bar
Flour tortilla	1 each
Waffle, frozen	4-inch waffle
Snack crackers	3–5 crackers
Muffin, small	1
10 GRAMS OF FAT*	Serving Size
Croissant	1
Waffle, homemade	7-inch waffle
Tabbouleh	1/2 cup

FRUITS	
1–2 Servings per Day	
NATURALLY CONTAIN LESS THAN 1 GRAM OF FAT	Serving Size
Citrus, berries, melons—daily for vitamin C	1 medium piece or 1/2 cup canned
Bananas or any other plain fruit	
Dried fruit	2 Tbsp. dried
Fruit juice (no sugar added)	1/2 cup juice

VEGETABLES	
4–5 Servings per Day	
NATURALLY CONTAIN 1 OR LESS GRAMS OF FAT*	Serving Size
Dark green leafy: leaf lettuce, greens, spinach, kale, broccoli, etc. Deep yellow/orange: carrots, winter squash, sweet potatoes**, tomato. Any other plain vegetable: corn, potato, cabbage, cauliflower, etc.	1/2 cup cooked or 1 cup raw
3–5 GRAMS OF FAT	Serving Size
Coleslaw	1/2 cup
Candied sweet potatoes	1/2 cup
Baked french fries	10 fries
Mashed potatoes	1/2 cup
10–15 GRAMS OF FAT*	Serving Size
Fried French fries	10 fries
Hashed brown potatoes	1/2 cup
Avocado	1/2 medium

SUGARS/FATS/DESSERTS	
Use Sugars in Moderation; Use as Little Added Fat as Possible	
0–2 GRAMS OF FAT*	Serving Size
Most sugars contain no fat but have no nutritional value other than calories. Blackstrap molasses** and full-fruit jams (no sugar added) do offer some vitamins and minerals in addition to the calories, so choose them more often than other sweeteners.	1 Tbsp. sugars or jam

*These are average grams of fat for food within each category.
**Nondairy foods high in calcium. If you do not consume dairy products, it is important to get several other good sources of calcium every day.

SUGARS/FATS/DESSERTS	
3–5 GRAMS OF FAT	Serving Size
Many desserts are high in fat and sugar; the following desserts contain less fat and sugar and some offer vitamins and minerals. Therefore, choose them more often than rich pies, cakes, cookies, ice cream, or candy	
Angel-food cake	1 med. slice
Graham crackers	2 long
Fig Newtons	2
Fat-free desserts	1–2 ounces
Ice milk, frozen yogurt, low-fat pudding	1/2 cup
Fruit-based desserts (cobbler or baked fruit)	1 piece
10 GRAMS OF FAT*	Serving Size
Use added fats sparingly, as they are concentrated in fat. Choose the polyunsaturated and monosaturated fats listed below, and limit intake of butter, stick margarine, shortening, coconut, sour cream, cream cheese, sausages, bacon, fried foods, chicken skin.	
Vegetable oils, olive, canola, safflower, sunflower, corn (5 grams fat)	1 tsp.
Soft tub margarine (5 grams fat)	1 tsp.
Mayonnaise (8–15 grams fat)	1 Tbsp.
Oil-based salad dressings (8–15 grams fat)	1 Tbsp.

ing fruit juice or a soda after exercise will replace needed water *and* carbs. If you are an endurance athlete, eating carbs after exercise is important in maximizing your glycogen stores. Any time you have worked your muscles to exhaustion, *carbohydrate recovery* is necessary. The average exerciser probably doesn't run out of glycogen in a typical exercise, but it is a good idea to *think carbs* after a workout anyway.

Tips for Weight Loss

There is absolutely no magic when it comes to losing weight. The magical quick fix does not last, so any quick and easy road to weight loss is also a quick and easy road to weight gain. Permanent weight loss only comes about through changing the behaviors that led to being overweight in the first place—i.e., overeating. Exercise and a low-fat, high-carbohydrate diet will help the body get rid of the excess body fat the

overeating caused. Here are some guidelines for designing a plan to manage your weight:

1. *Eat when you are hungry, and stop when you are satisfied.*

When not hungry, do something else. This is easy to say, but hard to do if you are used to skipping meals and then overeating in the evening. Some people have the false belief that they will eat fewer total calories if they skip a meal. Others say eating breakfast makes them more hungry during the day. Well, it is normal to get hungry sometime during the morning and at least two other times during a twenty-four hour period. Skipping meals sets up the urge to overeat. There is nothing wrong with eating three to six times a day. In fact, there is some indication that eating small, frequent meals can aid weight loss. So, if you are hungry, eat—regardless of how much you weigh!

2. *Set a realistic goal and then plan to take it slow, losing no more than one to two pounds per week.*
Instead of drastically cutting calories, pay attention to the amount of fat grams you are eating. Cut calories only by two hundred to five hundred per day and do several long, slow aerobic workouts a week. Diets lower than twelve hundred calories may give quicker results, but those results are usually temporary. Your body responds to a big drop in calories by decreasing its metabolic rate (energy output). Exercise helps to offset this drop, but you can't exercise very long on twelve hundred calories a day. Generally, I recommend women go no lower then fifteen hundred calories and men no lower than eighteen hundred calories per day. Otherwise, you need to be under the care of a dietitian or physician who specializes in weight management.

3. *Weigh only once a week at the most.*
Everyone experiences fluid shifts that can affect body weight temporarily. There is no point letting a one-pound water gain destroy your confidence in losing weight. Also, if you are exercising with weights as well as doing aerobic workouts, you will gain muscle weight at the same time you lose fat weight. But the scale cannot tell you that your body is getting leaner even though it may not have lost much weight. Rely on how

you feel and how your clothes fit to determine if you are making progress.

4. *Don't deprive yourself of foods you really want.*
If you make your diet too rigid—no sweets, for example—you will find yourself craving *forbidden* foods more than ever. To manage cravings, eat whenever you are hungry, choose well-balanced meals most of the time, and allow yourself to eat your favorite foods in reasonable portions. Taking away the *forbiddenness* of food eliminates the guilt associated with eating. Guilt is something that not only makes you feel bad, it often drives you right into the kitchen!

5. *Drink plenty of water.*
People sometimes avoid water thinking it will help them lose weight. Not true! In fact, avoiding water can force your body to hang on to as much fluid as possible, meaning it would actually retain water. If you do not drink enough liquids, your body will act like a cactus and store as much water as possible to prevent dehydration. So, drinking enough water actually helps weight loss by normalizing fluid balance.

6. *Periodically, write down everything you eat, when you eat, and why you eat.*
Recording this information will help you stay on track because it forces you to really pay attention to what goes in your mouth. It can help you identify times you are eating when you are not hungry. If you are eating because you are lonely or worried, food is not really what you need. You need company or a method to solve the problems that worry you. Eating during those times constitutes *overeating*. The overeating is what gets in the way of weight loss. You will need to find other ways to cope with the stresses of life. Exercise helps. Deep breathing exercises, calling a friend, writing in a journal, and taking a hot bath are other ways to manage stress.

7. *Don't expect yourself to be perfect.*
You aren't! If you overdo it with food or underdo it with exercise, forgive yourself and forget it. Take each day as it comes and do the best you can. Some days are easier than others. Focus on all the things you do right, not the things you do wrong. Beating yourself up about setbacks will only make you feel like a failure. You will give up, thinking, Oh well, what's the use? I'll never be thin so I might as well eat. A setback does not have to spell disaster unless you let it.

8. *Celebrate your success!*
Reward yourself for eating well and exercising because those are the behaviors that will help you sustain weight loss. But do not use food as the reward. Treat yourself in other ways—short trips, books, or anything that makes you feel good about yourself.

9. *Buy clothes that fit and look nice.*
Get rid of your *fat clothes* so you have nothing to grow back into. Live as though you planned to stay thinner. You should also get rid of the *thin clothes* you purchased after your last starvation diet. Those clothes may represent a body weight that is unrealistic for you to maintain. Seeing them in the closet will only remind you of what you can never be, instead of the healthy person you are. It is time to give up any unrealistic dreams of maintaining a body weight that is too low for you. Sustaining a *healthy* weight is more important than being skinny.

10. *Live now as though you had already reached your weight goal.*
Some people wait to fulfill their dreams until they are thin, only to find out being thin does not automatically make life wonderful. The things in life that make it wonderful can be had at any weight. Whether it is travel, seeking a relationship, or changing careers, living your dreams is not dependent on what you weigh. It may seem like you have to look good in a bikini before going to the Caribbean, but the water doesn't get any bluer just because you get thinner. Sure, everyone wants to be attractive, and today's definition of attractive is *thin*. But life is about more than being thin. If you learn to enjoy yourself now, losing weight and keeping it off will be much easier.

A DAY IN THE LIFE MEAL PLANNER

The following planner will help you organize your meals to fit your lifestyle and workout schedule. This meal planner is only a sketch to help you see your day. You will need to fill in the details to create your individual picture. Use the recipes that follow to help plan your day. The following two plans are designed around your training schedule: morning or evening.

3,000 CALORIE BREAKDOWN OF A SAMPLE DIET

The following sample diet suggests that you eat two larger meals and one lighter meal, along with your snacks.

2 big meals: 1,000 calories each = 2,000
1 light meal: 500 calories
2 snacks: 250 calories each = 500
Total = 3,000

Key Elements to Keep in Mind

1. Size of your meal or snack = the number of calories
2. Composition = the percentage of carbohydrates, proteins, and fats
3. Time = how long before or after your workout

MORNING WORKOUT

Preworkout Snack

Before you train in the morning you should have something light: juice, fruit, a smoothie, half a bagel or muffin, coffee/tea (optional). It is best to keep this snack primarily liquid since you'll probably be having it close to training time.

Workout: 6 to 8 A.M.

Keep hydrated with water or a workout drink.

Post-workout Breakfast

After training you need to replace your glycogen (stored energy) supplies with a primarily high carbohydrate breakfast (approximately 70 percent carbohydrates, 20 percent protein, and 10 percent fat).
Examples:
Pancakes or waffles
Oatmeal or breakfast cereal
Juice
Banana

Lunch

For lunch you need a balanced meal consisting of approximately 45 percent carbohydrates, 40 percent protein, and 15 percent healthy fats.
Examples:
Pasta with tuna fish or rice and beans burrito
Water

Dinner

Eat a balanced dinner consisting of approximately 45 percent carbohydrates, 40 percent protein, and 15 percent healthy fats.
Examples:
Salad
Baked potato
Grilled chicken breast

EVENING WORKOUT

Breakfast

Eat a balanced meal consisting of approximately 45 percent carbohydrates, 40 percent protein, and 15 percent healthy fats.
Examples:
Egg whites
Potatoes
Toast
Juice
Coffee (optional)
Water

Lunch

For lunch you need a balanced meal consisting of approximately 45 percent carbohydrates, 40 percent protein, and 15 percent healthy fats.
Examples:
Turkey sandwich with lowfat Swiss cheese
Baked tortilla chips and salsa
Carrot cake
Water

Preworkout Snack

Approximately an hour before working out.
It is important to make sure your blood sugar levels are high and your body is sufficiently hydrated before you workout. This snack could be a piece of fruit, yogurt, juice, or a manufactured preworkout drink.

Workout: 6 to 8 P.M.

Keep hydrated with water or a workout drink.

Dinner

After training you need to replace your glycogen supplies with a primarily high carbohydrate dinner (approximately 70 percent carbohydrates, 20 percent protein, and 10 percent healthy fats).
Examples:
Pasta with marinara sauce
Salad
Bread
Water

It is important that you consume a healthy, well-balanced diet consisting of fruits, vegetables, grains, legumes, and lean protein sources. This goes for your snacks also. Your snack is an opportunity to fill your body with a healthy energy source. Don't think of a snack as a chance to fill your body with junk food. Depending on your diet (especially if you're vegetarian) you may need to include a protein supplement in your diet.

Power Nutrition Recipes

The following recipes will get you started on a balanced, healthy diet.

APPLE-RAISIN OATMEAL

Makes 1 large serving

1   cup apple juice
2   tablespoons raisins
$^1/_2$ cup rolled oats

In a small saucepan, bring the apple juice and raisins to a boil. Stir in the oats. Cook, stirring often, until the oats are done, 3 to 5 minutes.

Nutritional information per serving: 325 calories, 7 gm protein, 70 gm carbohydrate, 3 gm fat, 11 mg sodium, 571 mg potassium, 47 mg calcium, 5 gm dietary fiber. Count as 3 fruit and 2 grain.

BAKED APPLE

Makes 2 servings
This recipe was modified from one in Joy of Cooking *by Irma Rombauer and Marion Becker (Bobbs-Merrill Company, 1975).*

2   large McIntosh or Jonathan apples
2   tablespoons sugar
$^1/_2$ teaspoon cinnamon
1 to 2 teaspoons low-fat margarine (I Can't Believe It's Not Butter Light works well)
4   tablespoons fat-free or low-fat granola

Preheat the oven to 375°. Wash the apples and remove each core to $^1/_2$ inch from the bottom. Remove the seeds. Combine the sugar and cinnamon. Fill the apple centers with the mixture. Dot the tops with low-fat margarine. Place the apples in a baking dish with $^3/_4$ cup boiling water. Bake for 30 minutes or until tender but not mushy. Top each apple with 2 tablespoons granola. Serve immediately.

Nutritional information per serving: 237 calories, 1.6 gm protein, 55 gm carbohydrate, 3 gm fat, 68 mg sodium, 284 mg potassium, 23 mg calcium, 5 gm dietary fiber. Each serving counts as 2 fruit, $^1/_2$ grain, and 1 sweet/sugar.

BLACK BEANS AND RICE

Makes 6 servings
This recipe was adapted from a recipe in New Recipes from Moosewood Restaurant *(Ten Speed Press, 1987).*

2   cups brown rice (yields 6 cups cooked)
Vegetable oil spray
1   tablespoon olive oil
1   medium onion, chopped
3   cloves garlic, minced
1   medium carrot, chopped
$^1/_2$ green bell pepper, chopped
$^1/_2$ teaspoon cumin
$^1/_2$ teaspoon coriander
1   tablespoon dried parsley
One 14.5-ounce can stewed tomatoes
Salt and pepper
Two 15-ounce cans black beans, drained
Fat-free sour cream or yogurt

Begin cooking the rice. Meanwhile, coat a large skillet with vegetable oil spray. Add the olive oil and sauté the onion and garlic for 3 minutes. Add the carrot and continue cooking for 3 minutes. Add the green pepper and sauté 5 minutes more. Add the spices, tomatoes (with juice), and salt and pepper to taste. Simmer until the vegetables are tender. Add the beans. Simmer 10 minutes more. Serve over the brown rice with fat-free sour cream or yogurt.

Nutritional information per serving (1 cup beans over 1 cup rice without sour cream): 376 calories, 13 gm protein, 72 gm carbohydrate, 4.6 gm fat, 120 mg sodium, 704 mg potassium, 77 mg calcium, 8 gm dietary fiber. Count as 2 ounces protein and 3 grain servings.

BREAKFAST BURRITO

Makes 1 large serving (or 2 small servings)

Vegetable oil spray
1   teaspoon canola oil
1   teaspoon minced garlic
$^1/_4$ cup chopped onion
1   small potato, cut into small chunks (about 1 cup)
$^3/_4$ cup egg substitute
1   tablespoon fresh cilantro (or $^1/_2$ tablespoon dried)

¹/₄ cup grated fat-free cheese
¹/₄ cup chunky salsa or Pico de Gallo (page 42)
2 flour tortillas
Salt and pepper

Spray a nonstick skillet with vegetable oil spray. Heat the canola oil and garlic over medium heat. Add the onion and potato. Cook, covered, over low to medium heat, turning occasionally, until potatoes are brown and tender. Pour the egg substitute over the potato mixture and continue to cook, stirring occasionally to break up the egg. When the egg is cooked, stir in the cilantro and cheese. Salt and pepper to taste. Top with salsa and serve with tortillas.

Nutritional information per recipe: 626 calories, 38 gm protein, 83 gm carbohydrate, 16 gm fat, 1290 mg sodium, 1440 mg potassium, 417 mg calcium, 5 gm dietary fiber. Count entire recipe, including tortillas, as 2 grain, 2 high carbohydrate vegetable, 1 low carbohydrate vegetable, 4 protein, and 1 fat.

"BETTER THAN EGG-A-MUFFIN"

Makes 1 serving

Vegetable oil spray
1 piece Wholesome and Hearty Garden Sausage (found in natural foods section)
1 egg
1 large bagel, toasted
1 tablespoon low-fat mayonnaise
2 large tomato slices
Salt and pepper

Spray a nonstick skillet with vegetable oil spray. Over medium heat, begin heating the sausage. After a couple of minutes, break the egg into the pan. Break the yolk. Cook the egg and sausage on both sides until done, about 5 minutes total. Spread the bagel with mayonnaise and make a sandwich using the sausage, egg, and tomato slices. Sprinkle with salt and pepper to taste.

Nutritional information per recipe: 448 calories, 19.5 gm protein, 68 mg carbohydrate, 10 mg fat, 661 mg sodium, 236 mg potassium, 239 mg calcium, 6 gm dietary fiber. Count as 4 grain, 1 protein, 1 low carbohydrate vegetable, and 1 fat.

EASY MICROWAVE FISH

Makes 5 portions, about 3.5 ounces each

1 pound fish fillets (orange roughy is especially good, or try sole)
¹/₂ teaspoon salt
¹/₄ teaspoon dill weed
¹/₈ teaspoon pepper (or to taste)
1 tablespoon chopped fresh parsley (or 1 teaspoon dried)
2 tablespoons lemon juice
1 tablespoon light margarine or light butter

Place the fish in a glass baking dish. Sprinkle the spices and lemon juice over the fish. Dot the fish with the margarine. Cover it with waxed paper and cook on high for 5 minutes or until the fish flakes with a fork. Let stand for 4 minutes before serving.

Nutritional information per 3.5 ounces: 95 calories, 17 gm protein, <1 gm carbohydrate, 2 gm fat, 302 mg sodium, 363 mg potassium, 38 mg calcium, 0 gm dietary fiber. Count each serving as 3 protein.

JICAMA STICKS

Makes 8 servings
This recipe, slightly modified, was discovered in Cuisine of the American Southwest by Anne Lindsay Greer, Harper & Row, 1983.

1 small-medium jicama
Several fresh limes
¹/₂ teaspoon chili powder (or paprika)
1 to 2 tablespoons fresh cilantro, chopped

Peel the jicama with a sharp knife and remove the fibrous, inner layer. Slice the white meat of the jicama into strips. Squeeze the lime juice over the jicama. Then sprinkle with the chili powder and cilantro.

Nutritional information is not available for this vegetable. Count as a low carbohydrate vegetable serving.

LOW-FAT HUMMUS

Makes 1³/₄ cups

2   15-ounce cans garbanzo beans (chickpeas) with juice
1   teaspoon sesame oil
5   tablespoons lemon juice (bottled or fresh)
2   teaspoons minced fresh garlic
¹/₄   teaspoon salt
¹/₂   teaspoon hot pepper sauce, such as Tabasco

Drain the beans and reserve the liquid. Blend the beans in a food processor. Gradually add the rest of the ingredients until smooth. Use the reserved liquid to thin the hummus, if needed. Consistency should be thick enough to spread on bread, but thin enough to eat as a dip.

Nutritional information per ¹/₂ cup: 128 calories, 6 gm protein, 21 gm carbohydrate, 3 gm fat, 144 mg sodium, 300 mg potassium, 38 mg calcium, 4 gm dietary fiber. Each ¹/₂ cup counts as 1 plant protein *or* 1 high carbohydrate vegetable

GRILLED TUNA

Makes 5 portions, 3.2 ounces each
This recipe was adapted from one by the National Fish and Seafood Council. I reduced the sodium content by using Worcestershire instead of soy sauce and omitting the salt.

1   pound fresh tuna, cut into 5 steaks

Marinade:
1   tablespoon lemon juice
2   tablespoons Worcestershire sauce
2   tablespoons orange juice
1   tablespoon tomato paste, no salt added
¹/₂   teaspoon minced garlic
¹/₂   teaspoon oregano
1   tablespoon chopped fresh parsley (or 1 teaspoon dried)
Pepper

Mix all ingredients for the marinade. Add the tuna, turning to coat well. Let the tuna stand at least 20 minutes in the marinade. Grill the fish for 5 minutes on each side, periodically basting with the marinade. Do not over-

cook, or the fish will be dry and tough. Note: Place the fish on a perforated pan on the grill to keep it from breaking apart when turning.

Nutritional information per serving: 179 calories, 27.5 gm protein, 3 gm carbohydrate, 6 gm fat (30 percent fat calories), 108 mg sodium, 396 mg potassium, 20 mg calcium, 0 gm dietary fiber. Count each serving as 3 ounces protein.

POACHED SALMON

Makes 4 servings, about 4 ounces each
This recipe is from a cookbook accompanying my Kenmore microwave.

1¹/₂   cups hot water
¹/₃   cup dry white wine
2   peppercorns
1   lemon, thinly sliced
1   bay leaf
1   teaspoon instant minced onion
1   teaspoon salt
2   large salmon steaks, about 8 ounces each

Pour the hot water and wine into a glass baking dish. Add the rest of the ingredients, except the salmon. Cook on high for 5 minutes, or until the water reaches a full boil. Carefully add the salmon steaks. Cover with plastic wrap or wax paper and cook on high for 2 to 3 minutes, until the fish becomes opaque. Let stand for 5 minutes to finish cooking. Discard the liquid. If desired, top with a small amount of plain yogurt mixed with dill weed or try Annie's No Fat Yogurt Dressing with Dill (found in natural foods section of grocery store).

Nutritional information for 4 ounces of salmon: 209 calories, 31 gm protein, 0 gm carbohydrate, 8.5 gm fat, 60 mg sodium, 516 mg potassium, 52 mg calcium, 0 gm dietary fiber. Count ¹/₂ salmon steak as 4 protein.

PICO DE GALLO

Makes 16 servings, ¹/₄ cup each
At my house, this dish goes quickly, so I always make a big batch. You may prefer to cut it in half. If the dish turns out too hot, dilute it with more tomato.

15 fresh jalapeño peppers
1   medium white onion

5   Roma tomatoes
4   tablespoons fresh cilantro (or to taste)
Pinch or two of salt

Wearing rubber gloves, carefully remove the stems and seeds from the peppers. (Depending on the peppers, this can be very hot and the seeds will only make it hotter. If you don't wear gloves, you will soon regret it!) Chop all the ingredients to a fine texture. An onion chopper or food processor is helpful, especially for the onions and peppers. However, the tomatoes can easily become too juicy, so chop them by hand. Gently mix all the ingredients. This dish should have very little juice; it isn't salsa. It is a wonderful condiment for eggs, fish, chicken, chili, and beans. You can use it in cooking or as a dip with fat-free tortilla chips.

Nutritional information per $1/4$ cup: 24 calories, 1 gm protein, 6 gm carbohydrate, <1 gm fat, 20 mg sodium, 216 mg potassium, 10 mg calcium, 1 gm dietary fiber. Count as 1 low-carbohydrate vegetable serving.

SWEET POTATO FRIES

Makes 3 servings of about 6 fries each
This recipe is from the cookbook Meals Without Squeals *by Christine Berman and Jacki Fromer (Bull Publishing, 1991).*

1   small sweet potato (about 12 ounces)
1   teaspoon vegetable oil (canola or safflower)
Salt (optional)

Heat an oven to 375°. Peel the sweet potato and cut it into sticks or wedges. Toss them with the oil in a bowl. Spread the sticks on a baking sheet and bake for about 30 minutes, turning them halfway through the cooking period. If desired, sprinkle with a little salt before eating.

Nutritional information per serving: 84 calories, 1 gm protein, 17 gm carbohydrate, 1.6 gm fat, 7 mg sodium, 240 mg potassium, 19 mg calcium, 2 gm dietary fiber. Count each serving, about 6 fries, as 1 high carbohydrate vegetable.

STIR-FRY CHICKEN AND VEGGIES

Makes 2 large servings
This recipe was inspired, in part, by Jane Brody's "Simple Tofu Stir-Fry," in Jane Brody's Good Food Book, *published by W.W. Norton, 1985.*

Sauce:
$1/4$ cup chicken or vegetable broth
1   tablespoon Worcestershire sauce
1   teaspoon lemon juice
1   tablespoon Mirin or dry sherry
6   ounces fettuccini noodles

Stir-Fry:
Pam or other nonstick cooking spray
1   teaspoon olive oil
1   teaspoon sesame oil (use chili oil if you like it really hot!)
1   tablespoon sesame seeds, preferably unhulled
1   tablespoon minced garlic
$1/2$ teaspoon crushed red pepper
6   ounces skinless chicken breast (or scallops)
2   carrots, sliced thin, on the diagonal
$1/2$ cup chopped onion
$1/2$ cup green peas, frozen
$1/2$ cup corn kernels, frozen
1   small zucchini, sliced thin

Mix together all sauce ingredients and set aside.

Cook the noodles in boiling water according to package directions. Meanwhile, coat a large nonstick skillet with cooking spray. Heat the olive and sesame oils over a medium flame. Add the sesame seeds, garlic, and red pepper. Sauté briefly and then add the chicken or scallops. Toss with the seeds and garlic to coat. Continue stirring while the chicken browns for about 2 minutes. Remove the chicken from the skillet and set aside.

Add the carrots and 2 tablespoons water to skillet. Reduce heat to low, cover, and cook until the carrots begin to soften, stirring occasionally. Remove the lid, add the onion, and cook, uncovered, 2 minutes more. Then add the peas, corn, and zucchini. Toss and cook for 1 minute. Then add the chicken and sauce. Toss all the ingredients well. Cover and cook until heated thoroughly, about 3 minutes. Serve over fettuccini noodles.

Nutritional information per $1/2$ serving: 646 calories, 43 gm protein, 91 gm carbohydrate, 12 gm fat, 344 mg sodium, 140 mg calcium, 895 mg potassium, 10 gm dietary fiber. Count each serving as 3 grain, 2 low carbohydrate vegetable, 1 high carbohydrate vegetable, 3 protein, and 1 fat.

QUINOA SALAD WITH MINT

Makes 7 servings, 1 cup each
This recipe is adapted from one created by the chefs at Al-falfa's, a grocery store in Boulder, Colorado. It is light and easy to prepare. I especially like it served with seafood.

1   cup dry quinoa (a South American grain sold in natural foods stores)
1   quart water
1/2 tablespoon salt
1   cup cucumber, diced (peel if waxed)
1/4 cup red onion, minced
1   cup celery, diced
2   tablespoons fresh mint, chopped
2   tablespoons fresh parsley, chopped
1   lime, juiced
2   tablespoons red vinegar
2   tablespoons extra virgin olive oil
Salt and pepper to taste

Rinse the quinoa according to the package directions. Bring the water and salt to a boil. Add the quinoa and cook for about 12 to 15 minutes. Drain the quinoa and let it cool. Prepare the other ingredients and mix them with the cooled quinoa. Serve chilled.

Nutritional information per cup: 142 calories, 6 gm fat, no cholesterol, 4 gm protein, 20 gm carbohydrate, 2 gm dietary fiber. Count 1 cup as 2 grain.

BLUEBERRY/STRAWBERRY CRUNCHY "MILK SHAKE"

Makes 1 large serving, about 2³/₄ cups
Makes a good recovery meal.

6   ounces plain fat-free yogurt
1   cup apple juice
3/4 cup frozen or fresh blueberries
3/4 cup frozen or fresh strawberries
1   to 2 tablespoons maple syrup
2   tablespoons low-fat granola

Blend all the ingredients together. Use half of the fruit frozen to make it cold and "milk-shake-like."

Nutritional information per recipe: 409 calories, 13 gm protein, 88 gm carbohydrate, 2.5 gm fat, 175 mg sodium, 1082 mg potassium, 421 mg calcium, 6 gm dietary fiber.

Count as 1/2 grain, 4 fruit, 1 milk/yogurt, and 1 sweet/sugar.

BREAKFAST BEANS

Makes 2 servings
1   can plain black beans
4   whole eggs
1/2 cup Pico de Gallo (page 42)
4   flour tortillas

Pour the beans, including juice, into a nonstick skillet. When the beans are slightly warm, carefully break the eggs over the top of the beans. Cover and cook on low-medium until the eggs are poached. Carefully scoop out half of the beans with 2 eggs on top. Top with half the Pico de Gallo and serve with warm tortillas.

Nutritional information per serving: 635 calories, 33 gm protein, 86 gm carbohydrate, 18 gm fat, 1509 mg sodium, 691 mg potassium, 125 mg calcium, 13 gm dietary fiber. Count half the recipe as 2 high carbohydrate vegetable, 1 low carbohydrate vegetable, 2 protein, and 2 grain.

EASY AND YUMMY BEANS

Makes about 4¹/₂ cups
1   pound dried beans (pinto or Anasazi are my favorites)
1   can Rotel tomatoes
2   canned or 1 fresh jalapeño pepper, cut into very small pieces
Fresh garlic or garlic powder to taste
1/8 cup chili powder (or more if you like)
Salt

Boil the beans in water for 3 minutes and let them soak for 8 hours or so. (This method of soaking will help reduce flatulence.) Drain and add fresh water to about 2 inches above the top of the beans. Add all remaining ingredients. Bring the mixture to a boil and then let simmer, covered, until done—usually takes 3 to 4 hours. Stir every so often and check the water level. Keep just enough water to keep the beans from burning. Add a little salt, if needed, after the beans are cooked.

Nutritional information per 1/2 cup: 85 calories, 5 gm protein, 17 gm carbohydrate, <1 gm fat, 124 mg sodium, 352 mg potassium, 40 mg calcium, 5 gm fiber. Count 1/2 cup as 1 plant protein *or* 1 high carbohydrate vegetable.

ZUCCHINI HEALTH MUFFINS

Makes 8 large muffins

2¼ cups whole wheat flour
¼   cup sugar
¼   cup nonfat milk powder
1   teaspoon cinnamon
¼   teaspoon salt
1   teaspoon baking soda
½   teaspoon baking powder
½   teaspoon ginger
1½ medium zucchini, shredded
8   ounces plain nonfat yogurt
¼   cup pure maple syrup
¼   unsweetened applesauce
½   cup nonfat egg substitute (such as Egg Beaters)
1   cup seedless raisins
1   teaspoon vanilla extract
Extra applesauce for garnish

Preheat an oven to 350°. Spray 8 large muffin cups with nonstick cooking spray. In a medium bowl, combine the first 8 ingredients. Stir thoroughly. In a large bowl, combine remaining ingredients. Mix thoroughly with a wire whisk. Add the flour mixture to the zucchini mixture, mixing just until the flour is moistened. Spoon the batter into the cups. Bake for 30 minutes or until a toothpick inserted in the center of each muffin comes out clean. Cool the muffins thoroughly on a wire rack before removing them from the muffin pans. Eat plain *or* slice and heat under a broiler; serve with additional applesauce.

These muffins are flavorful, almost fat-free, and not as sweet as traditional zucchini muffins. To make them sweeter, use nonfat vanilla yogurt instead of plain or use additional sugar instead of the nonfat milk powder.

Nutritional information per muffin: 254 calories, 9 gm protein, 57 gm carbohydrate, 0.8 gm fat (3 percent fat calories), 228 mg sodium, 502 mg potassium, 128 mg calcium, 5.7 gm dietary fiber. Count each large muffin as 1 grain and 1 sweet/sugar.

SPINACH OMELETTE

Makes 1 serving

Nonstick cooking spray
1   green onion, chopped (optional)
2   cups fresh spinach, torn into small pieces
½   cup Egg Beaters or other fat-free egg substitute (You can use 1 whole egg and 2 egg whites. This adds 5 grams of fat.)
Pinch of salt, pepper to taste
4   tablespoons fat-free or low-fat shredded cheese, any flavor

Coat a small, nonstick skillet with cooking spray. Over low-medium heat, cook the onion and spinach, covered, until the spinach is partially wilted, about 3 minutes. Pour the egg substitute over and around the spinach, covering the bottom of the skillet. Add pepper to taste and a pinch of salt. Cook on low until almost done. Sprinkle the cheese on top and continue to cook until the egg is set. To *finish* the omelette, either fold it in half and press it lightly to be sure all the egg is cooked *or* cook it under a broiler for a few minutes. Note: If you cook the egg with the lid on, it cooks fast and needs no *finish* step; however, the egg has a steamed flavor.

Nutritional information per recipe: 135 calories, 17 gm protein, 10 gm carbohydrate, 3.5 gm fat, 400 mg sodium, 747 mg potassium, 252 mg calcium, 2 gm dietary fiber. Count as 2 low carbohydrate vegetable and 3 protein.

SHRIMP COWPOT

Makes 4 servings

Vegetable oil spray
1   tablespoon garlic, minced
1   small onion, chopped (about 1 cup)
1   tablespoon canola or olive oil
½   teaspoon lemon grass
½   teaspoon cumin
¼   teaspoon crushed red pepper
¼   teaspoon fennel seeds
¼   teaspoon salt
Pepper to taste
3   large carrots, sliced on the diagonal (about 2 cups)
1   bell pepper, chopped
1   small can (7 ounces) tiny shrimp, drained
2⅔ cups cooked brown rice (about 1 cup raw)
Soy sauce (optional)

Spray a large nonstick skillet with vegetable oil spray. Over medium heat, sauté the garlic and onion in the oil. When the onions are translucent, add the spices and carrots; reduce the heat. Cook, covered, until the carrots are just tender, about 5 minutes. Add the green pepper and cook until all the vegetables are tender. Add the shrimp and rice. Stir together and heat through. Season with soy sauce to taste, if desired.

Nutritional information per serving, without soy sauce: 300 calories, 12 gm protein, 52 gm carbohydrate, 6 gm fat, 237 mg sodium, 509 mg potassium, 75 mg calcium, 6 gm dietary fiber. Count $1/4$ of recipe as 2 grain, 2 low carbohydrate vegetable, 1 protein, 1 fat.

PUMPKIN YOGURT

Makes 1$^1/_4$ cups

8   ounces vanilla fat-free yogurt
$^1/_2$ cup canned pumpkin

Combine ingredients.

Nutritional information per recipe: 203 calories, 9.4 gm protein, 42 gm carbohydrate, 0 gm fat, 111 mg sodium, 608 mg potassium, 283 mg calcium, 4 gm dietary fiber. Count entire recipe as 1 high carbohydrate vegetable, 1 milk/yogurt, and 1 sweet/sugar.

TANYA'S FROZEN YOGURT

Makes 1 large serving
My good friend Tanya Evtuhov shared this wonderful treat with me.

$^3/_4$ cup frozen, unsweetened blueberries (or any other
       unsweetened, frozen fruit)
$^3/_4$ cup nonfat, vanilla yogurt

Using a blender, thoroughly mix the fruit and yogurt. Eat right away or store in an airtight container in the refrigerator. Absolutely wonderful! Note: If you need to cut down on sweets, make this with artificially sweetened yogurt and save the carbohydrate and calories found in the sugar.

Nutritional information per serving: 219 calories, 8.5 gm protein, 46 gm carbohydrate, 0.7 gm fat, 106 mg sodium, 413 mg potassium, 259 mg calcium, 3 gm dietary fiber. Count as 1 fruit, 1 milk/yogurt and 1 sweet/sugar.

Common Questions About Nutrition and Exercise

Q: Now that I am exercising. do I need to take vitamin supplements?

A: That depends on how well you are eating. If you follow the Power Nutrition guidelines 90 percent of the time—say six out of seven days—you probably do not need supplements. Virtually all vitamins are involved, either directly or indirectly, in supporting an exercising body, especially the B vitamins. Exercisers tend to eat more calories and, consequently, more vitamins as well. If you are eating plenty of nutrient-dense, high-carbohydrate foods—whole grains, vegetables, legumes, and fruits—you are likely getting the B vitamins and other nutrients you need. However, if you have cut your calorie intake to fifteen hundred per day or less, your vitamin intake may not be adequate. Take a multiple vitamin/mineral supplement that provides 100 percent of the RDA (Recommended Dietary Allowance) for all nutrients. Other people who may need vitamin/mineral supplements are:

- those with exceptionally high nutrient needs (pregnant women)
- those who limit their intake of certain foods due to allergies or intolerances
- those who follow a strict vegan diet—no animal products. They may not eat enough vitamin B_{12}, riboflavin, and vitamin D.

Q: I take a multiple vitamin/mineral supplement, but it doesn't contain much calcium. Should I take calcium separately?

A: Calcium is a very bulky nutrient, so most multiple supplements only include about 10 percent of the RDA. If you include no milk, yogurt, or cheese in your diet, you may need extra calcium. However, there are other food sources of calcium. Check your Power Nutrition guidelines for nondairy foods high in calcium, and choose several of those daily.

Q: I try to eat well every day and take a vitamin supplement for added insurance. Is this okay?

A: Probably. Most multiple vitamin/mineral supplements are safe. But you do need to *avoid* taking megadoses of certain nutrients, especially vitamins A and D. A *megadose* is usually defined as being more than five times the RDA for vitamins A and D, and more than ten times the RDA for other nutrients. Large doses of nutrients can have a druglike affect in the body and should be taken only under the advice of a physician. Also, unless you are sure you need them, do not take single nutrients in large doses, as you may inadvertently create an imbalance with other nutrients. If you take supplements, be sure you need them and get advice from your physician or dietitian about how much to take.

Q: Since my body needs extra protein for bodybuilding, should I be taking a protein supplement?

A: It is true that exercisers, including bodybuilders, have a higher requirement for protein than nonexercisers. But that requirement is easily met with food. There is absolutely no proof that taking excess protein is an advantage for bodybuilders. Excess protein is either converted to fat or burned for energy; it is not converted to muscle.

There are some practical reasons, however, for using protein powder instead of food to meet part of your protein needs. Suppose you want to make a fruit shake with a little protein for a pre-exercise meal. You are allergic to milk, and raw eggs are not considered safe. (They carry a risk of salmonella poisoning.) Protein powder is a reasonable alternative. Also, most protein powders contain no fat, whereas eggs and most meats contain some fat. So, if you have a hard time getting enough protein without getting too much fat, protein powders can be useful. Keep in mind, though, protein powders may not contain other nutrients found in high-protein foods, and they are very expensive compared to food. If you can eat a varied diet that includes cooked egg whites and nonfat dairy products, you will not need to buy expensive protein supplements. Use them if you need to, but know that they offer no magic for building muscle.

Q: Is it true that amino-acid supplements have the same effect as steroids but are safer?

A: No. The usefulness and safety of amino-acid supplements are far from proven. The research in this area is incomplete, leaving many unanswered questions. The claims for amino acids are often based on research in people with various disease conditions or nonexercisers. What little research that has been done on athletes has not explored the effects of taking selected amino acids on other amino acids in the body. They are very expensive, and the doses are often too small to have any special effect anyway. Remember, when it comes to supplements, it is far easier to sell them than it is to research them.

Q: What are *metabolic enhancers*?

A: There are various products on the market that claim to help you burn fat or improve athletic performance in some way. These claims are generally unfounded. They are based on thinking that if compound *X* is involved in a certain metabolic job, taking it in high doses will speed up that metabolic task. This is not necessarily true. The body has many safeguards to regulate metabolism within normal limits. Anything that alters normal metabolism beyond normal parameters is a drug. Drugs have side effects and should be monitored by a physician.

At best, such supplements are harmless, with limited effectiveness. At worst, they can produce deficiencies in other nutrients or produce uncomfortable and dangerous side effects. The supplement industry is big business. If some of the money can be used to fund good research, perhaps we will find uses for some of these products. Until then, *buyer beware.*

Q: If most supplements don't work, why are there so many on the market?

A: Everyone wants something for nothing. Athletes will do just about anything to gain the competitive edge. They are ripe for *magical* products that can make them faster, stronger, or bigger. Regulation of such products is limited, and the FDA is just now beginning to take a closer look at nutritional supplements.

I believe there are good reasons for letting consumers take supplements even if they are not proven to work—freedom of choice, for example. On the other hand, consumers should be protected from false advertising and dangerous products. The supplement wars between government and manufacturers are just beginning. In the meantime, focus on working out and eating well to get the results you want. No supplement is a substitute for those.

Q: Will fasting make me healthier?

A: Fasting is touted as being necessary to *cleanse the body of toxins*. This doesn't make sense to me. Don't you think an organism as complex as the human body would have a built-in cleansing system? Well, it has several. The liver can destroy toxins or remove them from circulation. The kidneys regularly filter the blood and eliminate toxins and waste products through the urine. Also, bowel movements serve to continuously clean the colon. When you get sick with vomiting or diarrhea, that is the body's way of getting rid of a poison in the gastrointestinal tract.

Fasting for more than twenty-four hours will rid your body of its glycogen stores and force you to convert protein (muscle) to blood sugar. You will lose weight rather quickly, but it is mostly water, glycogen, and protein, not fat. Fasting for more than three days makes you feel light and *high*. There can be spiritual benefits from foregoing food for several days, but nutritionally, fasting is not necessary or even helpful.

Q: Some of my friends take diuretics to look more muscular. Are they safe?

A: Many bodybuilders use diuretics to enhance the *cut* of their muscles before a competition or photo session. Diuretics force the kidneys to excrete water that is normally found in muscles and other parts of the body. They do temporarily make you look thinner or more muscular. However, the body does not function well in a dehydrated state. It can be very dangerous to take diuretics on a regular basis. Waste products build up in the body, causing damage to various organs. The only reason you should take a diuretic is if you have an *abnormal* buildup of fluid. Even the mild nonprescription diuretics can be dangerous if abused. Your healthiest bet is to stay away from them unless they are recommended by your physician.

Q: Is it true that caffeine will help me burn more body fat?

A: Caffeine increases the amount of fatty acids in the blood and the use of fat for energy during exercise. Some research reports that exercisers can run longer with caffeine than without. The dose used was equivalent to drinking two to three cups of brewed coffee one hour before exercising. However, consuming caffeine may offer no advantage over that of consuming a high-carbohydrate diet to maximize glycogen stores.

People vary in their tolerance to caffeine, a stimulant found in coffee, tea, cocoa, cola beverages, and some medications. It may make you feel great, or it may make you a nervous wreck. Caffeine is also a diuretic. If you drink coffee or tea before exercising, you may find yourself having to interrupt your workout to go to the bathroom.

In moderation—say, two cups of coffee per day—caffeine is safe for healthy adults. Its benefits may be more perceived than real, but if you have no negative side effects, go ahead and try it if you want. Large doses of caffeine (amounts equal to eight cups of coffee) have been banned by the U.S. Olympic Committee.

Summing It Up

Feeding your body well offers numerous benefits. You will be more energetic, feel better, and perhaps prevent or delay illness. Good nutrition cannot guarantee you will develop the body shape you desire, but it goes a long way in helping you meet your full potential for a healthy, fit body. Eating to support exercise will give your body an extra push when it is most needed. Eating to support life will pay off in all your endeavors. *Bon appétit!*

CHAPTER SIX

Lower-Back Basics

by BRYON HOLMES, M.S.

You are in a privileged and small minority, if you don't suffer from lower-back pain. Low-back pain will cause 80 percent of all Americans to miss at least one week of work during their lifetime. It is the most expensive health-care cost in America. Eighty billion dollars a year can be directly attributed to low-back problems.

The Unguarded Moment

Ninety percent of all low-back pain may be attributed to soft tissue. Soft tissue refers to muscle, tendon, and ligaments. Most low-back injuries occur during an "unguarded moment." This moment occurs when an individual has to suddenly react to his or her environment. Injuries also occur when an individual turns, twists, stoops, or bends in an unusual manner. Picking up light objects and sneezing are common examples of unguarded moments. It is not the object or sneezing that caused the pain, but years of soft-tissue deconditioning.

Acute and Chronic Pain

Back pain can be categorized into two phases: acute pain and chronic pain. Back pain is considered acute during the first six weeks. Most low-back pain (80 percent) will resolve itself within six weeks regardless of the intervention. This explains why the most common medical advice during the acute phase is to rest and take anti-inflammatory medication.

When back pain continues beyond six weeks, it is considered chronic. When an individual is suffering from low-back pain, his or her natural reaction is to splint or guard any movements that require the back to work. This will temporarily prevent the back musculature from being exposed to external forces. This relieves short-term pain, but the long-term effects can be devastating. Pain leads to disuse; disuse leads to muscular atrophy; atrophy leads to weakness. Weakness predisposes an individual to pain because of the inability to withstand normal usage. This continuous cycle is referred to as the *chronic deconditioning syndrome.* Chronic disuse atrophy or the deconditioning syndrome can be compared to an individual who has an arm in a cast for six to eight weeks. After removal of the cast, an obvious weakness in muscle strength is apparent. The human body physiologically adapts to the demands placed upon it. The muscle group in question has essentially adapted to no stimulation, by allowing unused muscle to atrophy and weaken.

Prevention

Weak muscles are a major contributing factor in back pain. Strength of the trunk extensors is reduced in the patient with chronic back pain. Adequate strength of the trunk muscles is necessary for a full return to function and work. It is quite possible to increase the functional and structural integrity of the low back by increasing the competency of the soft tissues. Most low-back pain is preventable and can be treated and managed successfully. You can increase a muscle's contractile ability (strength) by exposing it to regular overload stimulation (strength training). In other words, by isolating and strengthening the muscles, you can treat and prevent back pain. Increasing your levels of strength increases your structural integrity and your ability to withstand the unguarded moment. Specific exercise is the only effective way to prevent low-back problems. It is also the only effective way to prevent and control the recurrence of chronic low-back pain once it has developed.

All movement, even sitting and maintaining an upright posture, requires the low-back muscles to work. The back muscles are the most important in controlling the mechanics of the spine. Everyday movements help to build and maintain a certain degree of low-back strength. Most strength gains, however, are achieved during a movement of trunk extension which occurs in the muscles that rotate the pelvis and not the lumbar spine.

The lumbar spine must be isolated during exercise to get stronger. During trunk extension, the hip flexors are the primary movers and the lumbar extensors are the secondary movers. If the lumbar extensors are to get strong, they must be isolated so they can be overloaded by being exposed to greater work loads than usual; then they become stronger and prepared to withstand the unguarded moment. At the present time, there is only one device on the market that will prevent pelvic rotation as the trunk extends—the MedX lower-back machine.

Lower Back and the ABs

The abdominals play an important and intricate role in the prevention and rehabilitation of the lower back. The lower back is not a unit in and of itself; it is part of the trunk. Imagine the trunk as a large barrel, inside of which are the body's essential organs. Barrels used in the fermentation process of winemaking have steel bands that wrap around them for support; the abdominal musculature acts like these steel bands, maintaining intra-abdominal pressure. Weak abdominal musculature allows the abdomen to sag, creating greater load on the low back, forcing it to hold up the mass in front of it. Strong abdominal musculature will prevent a forward sag and keep stress off the low back.

Strengthening ABs creates greater intra-abdominal pressure; increased pressure forces a more upright positioning of the spine. The net result is a decreased load on the lumbar disks. Reducing this load will decrease the likelihood of having a ruptured or slipped disk. Poor posture contributes to low-back pain. Increasing the strength of the lumbar extensors and the ABs will help to improve posture, decreasing the incidence of back pain. Strong lower-back muscles and strong ABs work together in maintaining a pain-free and healthy back.

Other Key Areas

HIPS AND BUTTOCKS The muscles of the buttocks and hips support and assist the lower back. Most movement involving the lower back also involves pelvic rotation. It is important to strengthen the muscles around the girdle (hips and butt) so they can help support the lower back. Exercises that are good for these areas are: lunges, leg press, body-weight squats, adduction and abduction movements. Check with a qualified fitness professional about how to do these.

UPPER BACK AND CHEST As stated earlier, good posture is essential to lower-back wellness. It is common, however, for there to be an imbalance between the chest and back. Because we tend to do everything in front of us, the chest and shoulders tend to be stronger than the back, causing the upper torso to roll forward and shifting the torso into a forward posture. To alleviate this and to align the spine correctly, it is important to exercise the upper back as much as (and in the beginning possibly more than) the chest. This will balance and center the torso, thereby improving posture.

HAMSTRING FLEXIBILITY Flexibility in the hamstrings (backside of thigh) is important to the lower back because the hamstrings attach into the hip area. The erector spine in the lower back also attaches into the hips. A tight hamstring will prohibit the range of motion of the erector spine, when one bends over (trunk flexion), thereby limiting its ability to gain strength. One must maintain flexibility in the hamstrings to avoid this. A good exercise for this is the hamstring stretch on page 60.

Low-back pain is usually caused by a combination of factors. If you have chronic low-back problems it is important that you work with a qualified professional to treat the problem holistically.

The Exercises and Program

The following exercises will help strengthen the muscles of your lower back. They are listed in order of difficulty. Choose an exercise that fits your fitness level and incorporate it into your ABs training. Do your lower back exercise at the end of your ABs routine.

BASIC GUIDELINES FOR BACK STRENGTHENING Always work within a range of motion in which you feel no pain. If it is painful to reach certain positions, then stop short of them during exercise. Exercises designed to increase strength will increase strength fifteen degrees beyond the end point of the movement. Therefore, stopping movement just prior to a position of discomfort will provide significant strengthening benefits beyond that range of motion. Never use a sudden movement when performing a strength exercise even though it is harder to do a slow, controlled movement. Sudden movements use momentum. By performing a slow, controlled movement, you will not be able to handle as much resistance, but muscular fatigue (overload) is still accomplished, and the risk of injury is greatly reduced.

LOWER-BACK EXERCISES

Opposite Arm and Leg—On Knees: Start on all fours, resting on your hands and knees. You should look straight down, neither tucked or looking up. From this position, simultaneously raise and straighten your right arm and left leg until they are parallel to the ground (or as close to parallel as you can) without going past the parallel position. Hold for two seconds and come back slowly to the starting position. Repeat with left arm and right leg. Start with ten repetitions on each side and build up to twenty repetitions.

Opposite Arm and Leg on Stomach—Facedown: Lie facedown on the floor, arms extended overhead, palms on the floor. From this position, simultaneously raise your right arm and left leg as high as you can comfortably. Hold for two seconds and come back to the floor slowly. Repeat with left arm and right leg. Build up until you can complete twenty repetitions easily.

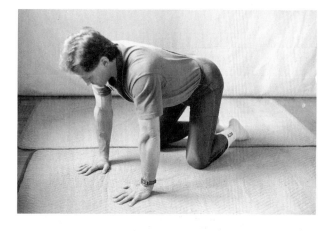

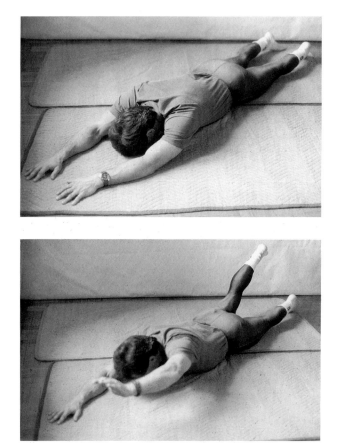

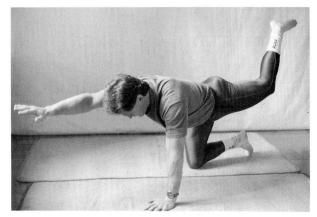

Basic Trunk Extension: Lie facedown flat on the floor, place your heels under a couch, leaving your arms at your sides. Slowly, raise your chest off the floor as high as you comfortably can. Hold for two seconds and come back to the floor slowly. Gradually increase until you can do twenty repetitions easily.

Intermediate Trunk Extension: Lie facedown with a firm pillow under your pelvis, place your heels under a couch, leaving your arms to your side. Slowly, raise your chest off the floor as high as you comfortably can. Hold for two seconds and come back to the floor slowly. When you can do twenty repetitions easily, place another pillow under your pelvis. This will increase the difficulty and range of motion of the exercise.

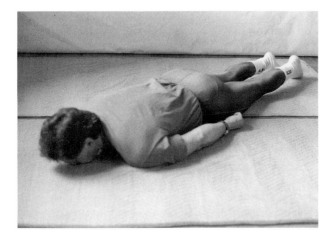

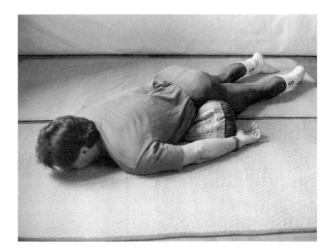

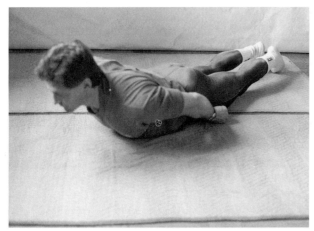

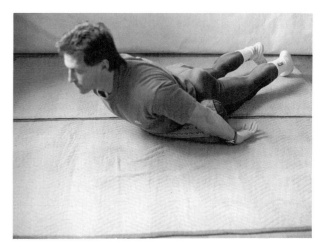

Advanced Trunk Extension: Lie facedown on a bed, table, or exercise bench. Have someone hold your ankles as you slide forward until your pelvis is on the edge of the table and your trunk is hanging off. Slowly, raise up as high as you can, hold for two seconds, and then come back down as far as possible. When you can accomplish twenty repetitions, start holding weighted objects in your hands as you do the exercise.

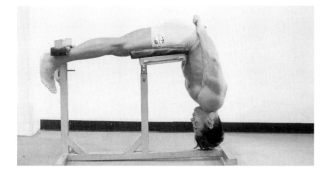

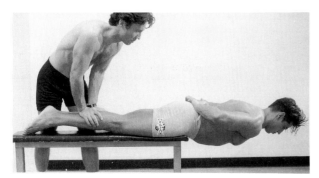

To the Core

The purpose of this routine is to work your power center. A strong power center will also help you overcome the "unguarded moment." The major muscles of the power center include the glutes (butt), the ABs, and the lumbar extensors. One or more of these muscles are used in almost every activity. This program was developed by Mike Brungardt to train professional athletes to sustain the rigors and punishment of a long season.

THE ROUTINE:

• Position 1—Face Up: Rest on your elbows (making a fist, thumbs up) and your heels, keeping your hips off the floor. Keep your body straight and stiff like a board.

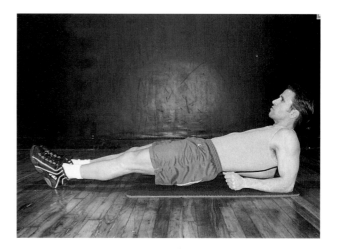

• Position 2—Left Side: Rest on your left elbow (making a fist, thumb up) and the outside of your left foot. Keep your forearm perpendicular to your body. Keep your hip off the floor. And keep your body straight and stiff like a board.

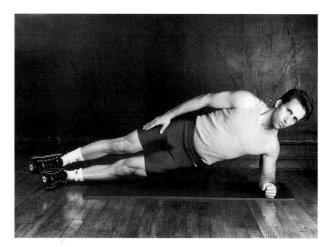

- Position 3—Face Down: Rest on your elbows (making a fist, thumbs up) and your toes, keeping your hips off the floor. Keep your body straight and stiff like a board.
- Position 4—Right Side: Rest on your right elbow (making a fist, thumb up) and the outside of your right foot. Keep your forearm perpendicular to your body. Keep your hip off the floor. And keep your body straight and stiff like a board.

GUIDELINES:

Start by holding each position for ten seconds, eventually work up to a one minute hold for each of the four positions.

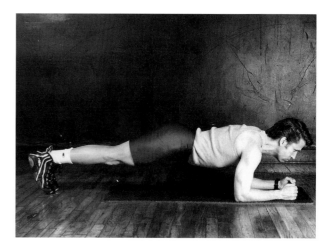

ABS WORK FOR THOSE WITH LOWER-BACK PROBLEMS If you have lower-back problems, you face special challenges when working out your Abs. It is important for you to start slowly and build gradually. You may feel that you can do more during the early phases, but remember it is quality, not quantity, that is important. If you skip to higher levels, you may not establish the base of strength necessary to achieve overall abdominal balance. You also may injure yourself. So start with the first level, and progress according to recommendations. Your lower-back problems didn't develop overnight. Your abdominal strength won't either. If you have lower-back problems, it is imperative that you check with a doctor before beginning an exercise program. When exercising, it is also important that you learn how to distinguish between good and bad pain, as discussed in Chapter 3. If you have a history of lower-back pain, you should *not* exercise through spasm, lingering pain, or shooting, peripheral pain.

Each exercise has a lower-back rating. Check it before choosing exercises. *Low risk* does not mean the exercise is guaranteed to be safe for your back. It means you are at a lower risk of injury. It is also important, when possible, to keep your lower back pressed against the floor when exercising. This gives your lower back support and prevents arching. You should also never jerk or perform sudden, extreme movements; always roll up and down your spine gently and gradually. You don't need to do the most advanced exercises to develop abdominal strength that will support your lower back and improve your posture. Once you have developed a solid base of strength, you may be able to move to more advanced exercises. Just remember to go slow and work with a doctor, physical therapist, or fitness trainer when in doubt.

The important thing to remember is, if you have a lower-back problem, part of the problem is low-back weakness. You have to strengthen the weak area. Proper stretching and specific lower-back exercises will help strengthen and prevent recurring back pain. If you take care of your back, it will last a lifetime.

On page 248, you'll find a specialized, progressive AB routine for low-back sufferers. It is specifically designed for those with lower-back pain; unless you have very serious problems, you should be able to do these exercises safely, but again, that's no guarantee you won't encounter difficulties. Everybody's lower back is different, and people's problems here vary widely. Only you and your doctor can determine what's right for your individual case. You should experiment very carefully. If any exercise causes "bad" pain, you should stop immediately.

CHAPTER SEVEN

The Complete Person: An Introduction

by DEBBIE HOLMES, M.S.

Abdominal development is an important part of physical well-being. Yet it is only one component of exercise wellness, just as your physical well-being is only a single part of overall wellness. This chapter will outline life beyond great ABs. It will introduce the six areas of wellness, emphasizing the key elements of exercise wellness.

What Is Wellness?

Complete wellness is a lifestyle. It centers around your ability to take responsibility for how you live and the choices you make. Wellness means taking an active role in improving every aspect of your life in order to achieve a productive, healthy lifestyle.

The Six Dimensions of Wellness

There are six major dimensions of wellness: physical, emotional, spiritual, intellectual, vocational, and social. The choices you make in developing these dimensions will reflect the type of lifestyle you lead. And being aware of these choices is your first step to change.

Physical development encourages all issues concerning your physical body. These include daily exercise, diet, and medical care. They also include the use and abuse of tobacco, drugs, and alcohol.

Emotional development emphasizes awareness and acceptance of your feelings. As an emotionally well person, you maintain satisfying relationships with others while feeling positive and enthusiastic about your own life. You also maintain minimal levels of stress, develop healthy feelings, and use nondestructive emotional outlets.

Intellectual development encourages creative, stimulating mental activities. An intellectually well person uses all resources and knowledge available to improve skills, while expanding potential for sharing with others. Intellectual stimulation is a form of growth for the human body. Learning is crucial in order to make changes in your lifestyle.

Social development encourages contributing to the human community and physical environment. A socially well person emphasizes interdependence with others, with nature, and within his or her own family. A socially well person has developed healthy ways to interact, react, and live with other people involved in his or her life.

Vocational development encourages growth and happiness in your work. A vocationally well person seeks jobs that give personal satisfaction and enrichment.

Spiritual development is the quest for meaning and purpose. A spiritually well person develops, evolves, and practices his religious, political, environmental, and personal beliefs.

To understand complete wellness, we should look at these dimensions as if they were part of a pie chart.

A pie chart is a circle divided into six even slices representing the six dimensions of wellness. Each piece of the pie is important to the whole. A complete pie chart with all the pieces fitting together shows a healthy wellness profile. If one piece of pie has a problem, it will affect all the other pieces.

For example, if you recently fell and broke your ankle, your physical wellness would be taxed. Because of this, it is likely that vocational wellness will suffer, if your job requires you to be active and/or you missed work due to your injury. Emotionally, you would also be stressed because of injury. And because of dependency on family and friends, your social component

would also be affected. Everything intermingles to create that web of wellness.

Everyone's Different

It's important to understand that not everyone's pie chart will look the same. For instance, a professor at a university may have a larger piece of pie for intellectual stimulation than a housewife, whose social and family interactions are more important. An athlete would have a larger piece of physical pie than a minister of a church, whose religious beliefs are the substance of his life. Each one of our pie charts will look different, with emphasis on the things that make us different.

Creating your wellness pie chart means looking into what is important to you. The divisions of your pie chart will directly reflect how much time and importance each of the six dimensions has for you. Look at dividing your chart on a percentage basis. Out of the 100 percent, how important are the different dimensions? For example: 30 percent importance on physical wellness, 20 percent importance on vocational wellness, 13 percent importance on social, 13 percent emotional, 13 percent intellectual, and 11 percent on spiritual wellness. It's difficult to place a numerical value on these dimensions, but this kind of introspection will lead to valuable self-knowledge.

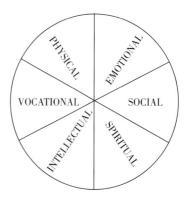

The Physical Dimension

Since this is a book about ABs, we will go into detail about physical well-being, specifically exercise wellness.

Just as you created your overall wellness profile, you can also develop a comprehensive program for "Physical Wellness." There are many benefits of exercise: stress reduction, weight loss, cardiovascular benefits, muscular strength, endurance, and increased flexibility. To achieve these benefits, however, you need a complete fitness program that works the four major areas of exercise wellness: cardiovascular, muscular strengthening, muscular endurance, and flexibility. The next chapter will outline basic workout programs that cover these areas.

CHAPTER EIGHT

Physical Wellness: Stretching, Cardiovascular, Lifting

The Program

It is important that you begin your comprehensive exercise program slowly and increase your exercise levels as you feel comfortable. Remember, the goal of physical wellness is to achieve a balance among all three components.

WARM-UP Before you start to exercise it is important to warm up. If you are at a gym, five minutes on the cardiovascular machine of your choice is a sufficient warm-up. If you are at home and you have a stationary bike, rower, or other cardiovascular machine, do the same. If not, a brisk five-minute walk is an excellent warm-up.

Stretching

Stretching works the muscles, ligaments, and joints. Flexibility is important in maintaining posture, joint mobility, and range of motion, and helps keep the ligaments and tendons from tightening. Stretching needs to be done at least three times a week and should involve all major muscle groups and joints.

A stretching routine should include stretches for all the primary muscles. It is important to begin and end your exercise program with stretching. Light stretching at the beginning of a workout is a good way to warm up your body. Stretching at the end of a workout is a good way to cool down and safely improve your flexibility when your body is warm.

You should start slow and stay within your comfort

zone. Stretch only until you feel slight discomfort (not pain!). Then hold that position without bouncing for the recommended time.

Knees-to-Chest Hug: Lie flat on your back, bring both knees to your chest. From this position, wrap your arms around your legs and hug your knees to chest. At the same time, bring your chin to your chest.   15 sec. × 2

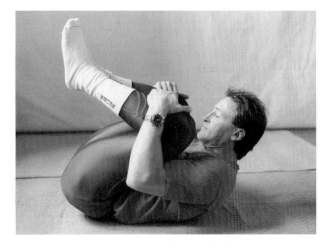

Hamstring: Lie on your back, legs bent, feet flat on the floor. Grab one leg behind your knee, straighten the leg, and gently pull it toward your head (chin to chest).   15 sec. × 2

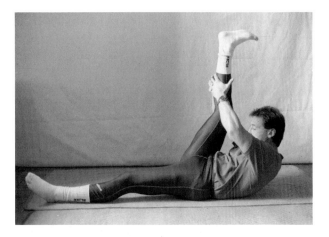

Knees to Side: Lie flat on your back, knees bent, feet flat on the floor.   Hold 10 sec.
Let both legs fall to one side. Then let the legs fall to the other side.   Hold 10 sec.

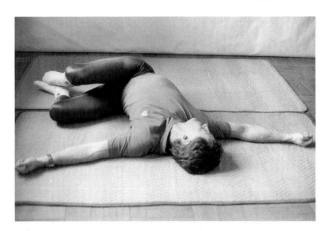

Elongation: Lie flat on your back, arms fully extended over your head, legs fully extended on the floor; extend from your finger tips to your toes, lengthening your body in both directions.   15 sec. × 2

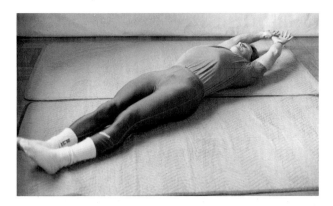

Back and Stomach: Lie on your stomach, hands under your chest (palms down). Slowly pressing up with your arms, straighten them as much as you can and arch your back. Relax lower body. Look up, attempting to get your chin as high as possible.   15 sec. × 2

Back Arch: Come up on your hands and knees (all fours).   15 sec. × 2

Place hands under your shoulders and hunch your back up like a cat and lower your head. Then arch your back in the opposite direction.   15 sec. × 2

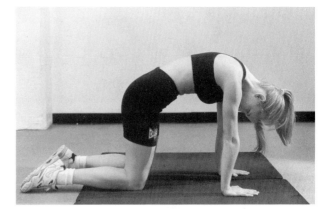

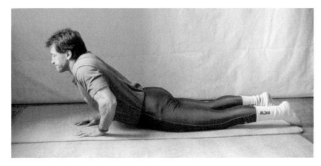

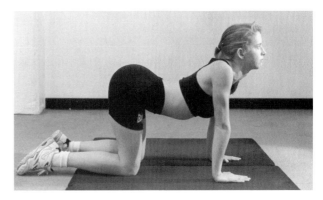

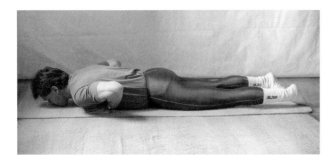

Quadriceps: Turn on one side and lie comfortably with shoulder under ear. Reach behind your back for your top ankle and gently pull it back. Then switch sides.   15 sec. × 2

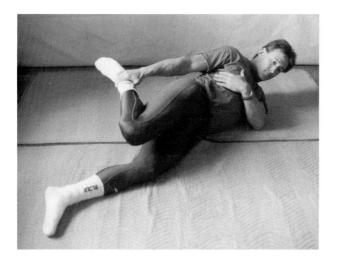

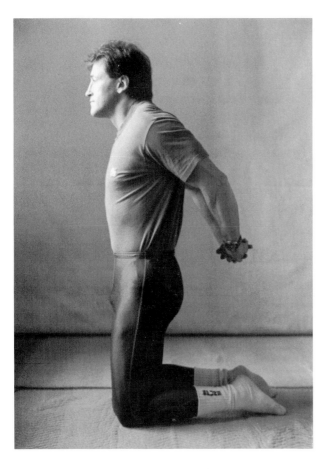

Chest: Kneeling erect, clasp your hands behind your lower back and slowly try to extend your hands up and back.   15 sec. × 2

Shoulders: Grasp hands in front of your body and turn palms forward while fingers remain interlocked; stretch shoulders forward, as you reach out as far as possible, rounding your back.   15 sec. × 2

Maintain hand position, stretch up, straight overhead.   15 sec. × 2

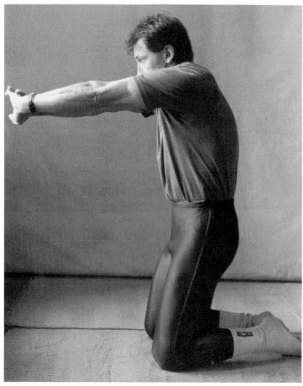

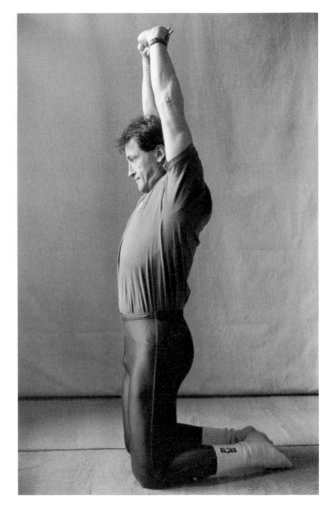

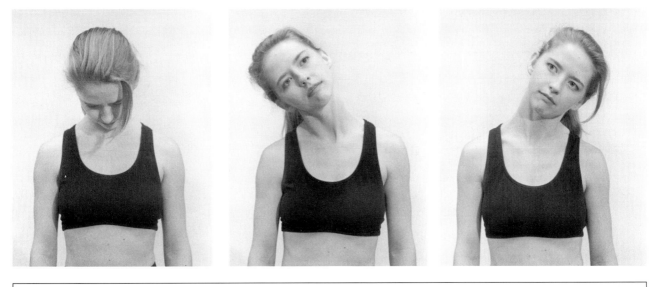

| **Neck:** Drop head forward, chin to chest. | 10 sec. hold | Lower your left ear to your left shoulder. | 10 sec. hold |
| Looking straight ahead, lower your right ear to your right shoulder. | 10 sec. hold | Turn head to both sides, looking as far back over each shoulder as possible. | 10 sec. hold |

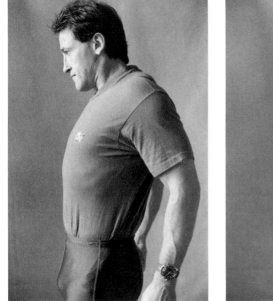
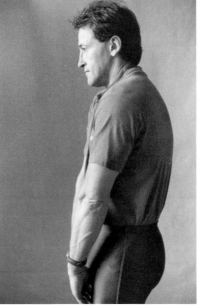
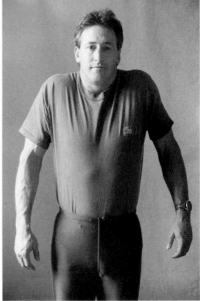

| **Shoulder Roll:** Standing, raise your shoulders high on your neck and roll them backward. | 5 reps. | Then bring your shoulders up toward your ears and hold for a count of ten and release. |
| Then repeat the movement, but roll your shoulders forward. | 5 reps. | |

Side Bend: Standing, feet together, arms fully extended over your head, hands touching. Bend at your waist over your right side.	10 sec.	Then bend at your waist over your left side.	Hold 10 sec.

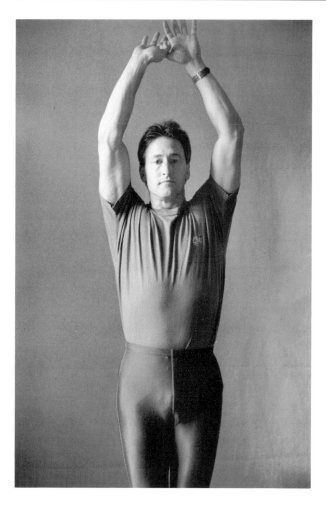 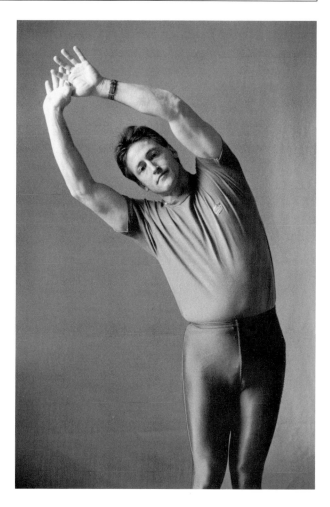

Cardiovascular (Walking, Jogging, Swimming, Cycling, Etc.)

Cardiovascular Fitness is achieved by performing activities that tax the heart, lungs, and circulatory systems. When cardiovascular exercise is performed, the body puts a demand on the oxygen-exchange systems of your body. Oxygen is taken from the lungs into the circulatory system, then distributed to the muscles that are being used during exercise. The oxygen is then used to help break down the stored fats into energy for the working muscle. This exchange system forces the lungs and heart to become extremely efficient, so that the working muscles can continue their activities.

The American College of Sports Medicine states that thirty minutes of cardiovascular exercise at least three times a week is sufficient to produce significant health benefits. A cardiovascular program consists of activities that allow you to reach 65–85 percent of your maximum heart rate for a duration of no less than twenty minutes. The kinds of exercises that we are discussing are walking, jogging, swimming, bicycling, aerobic dancing, etc. Maintaining these kinds of exercises longer than twenty minutes may provide additional benefits if the exercises are performed correctly.

FINDING YOUR TARGET HEART RATE

The following formula will determine your target heart rate for doing cardiovascular work. The following example is for someone who is thirty years old.

At birth your maximum heart rate is 220 beats per minute. Each year you age, your maximum heart rate decreases by one beat. So to determine your maximum heart rate, you subtract your age from 220.

For training purposes, you want to achieve between 65 and 85 percent of your maximum heart rate, so to figure out what your ten-second pulse rate should be, divide your maximum heart rate (220 minus your age) by .65 and .85, and then divide those figures by 6 (because there are 6 ten-second periods in every minute). The two resulting figures are the low and high ends for your ten-second pulse during training. When working out, you want to keep your heart rate between these parameters.

$$220 - 30 = 190 \text{ beats per minute}$$
(Maximum heart rate)

$$190 \times .65 = 123.5 \text{ beats per minute}$$
(Lower end of target)

$$190 \times .85 = 161.5 \text{ beats per minute}$$
(Upper end of target)

To figure out the target ten-second pulse:

Divide your upper and lower target numbers by 6. These are your upper and lower target pulses for ten seconds during exercise.

In the middle of your exercise session, count your number of heartbeats in ten seconds by checking your pulse at your wrist or on your neck. It should be somewhere between the upper and lower ends of your target pace. So in the example above, you want to be between twenty-one and twenty-seven beats in the ten count.

Cardiovascular Program: The following are general guidelines for a progressive cardiovascular program.

Weeks 1 and 2:	5-minute easy pace
	5-minute *target* pace
	5-minute easy pace
	15 minutes' total time
Weeks 3 and 4:	5-minute easy pace
	5-minute *target* pace
	2-minute easy pace
	5-minute *target* pace
	5-minute easy pace
	22 minutes' total time
Weeks 5 and 6:	5-minute easy pace
	10-minute *target* pace
	2-minute easy pace
	10-minute *target* pace
	5-minute easy pace
	32 minutes' total time
Weeks 7 and 8:	5-minute easy pace
	15-minute *target* pace
	2-minute easy pace
	15-minute *target* pace
	5-minute easy pace
	42 minutes' total time
After 8 weeks' Maintenance:	
	5-minute easy pace
	10–30-minute *target* pace
	5-minute easy pace
	20–50 minutes' total time

Lifting (Strength Training)

Strength Training provides increased strength gains and increased endurance for the muscles, joints, bones, and ligaments of the body. The kind of benefits achieved with strength training include developing a better posture and stronger structural features, stronger bones, increased strength for daily activities, good muscle tone, flexibility and strength in joints.

Strength training should include exercises designed for all major muscle groups of the body, and should be performed at least two to three times per week. Strength training can be done a variety of ways: free weights, strength machines, or through other resistive kinds of training methods. There are a variety of strength-training programs that will help you to achieve all the possible physical benefits.

Your strength-training program needs to include exercises for all muscle groups. You should train larger muscle groups first, followed by your smaller muscles.

If you are unfamiliar with these exercises, it is important that you consult a qualified professional.

EXERCISES TO CHOOSE FROM:

Back
Pullovers
Upright Rows
Bent-over Rows
Single-Arm Rows
Lat Pulldowns *(behind the neck)*
Lat Pulldowns *(to the chest)*
Rear Flys
Low-Back Extensions

Legs
Leg Extensions *(Quadriceps)*
Leg Curls *(Hamstrings)*
Squats
Lunges
Calf Raises

Chest
Bench Press
Flat Bench Flys
Incline Bench Press
Incline Flys
Pullovers
Wide-Arm Push-ups

Triceps
Tricep Extensions
Overhead Extensions
Tricep Kickbacks
Close-Grip Bench Press
Dips
Close-Grip Push-ups

Shoulders
Lateral Raises
Overhead Press
Front Raises
Rear Flys

Biceps
Straight Curls
Individual Curls

Concentration Curls
Hammer Curls

Extras to Add Side Bends
Neck Exercises
Wrist Curls

When beginning your program, be sure to choose a weight that will allow you to reach a point of fatigue within a reasonable number of repetitions. You need to determine repetition goal each time you exercise, so write down the number of repetitions you do after each exercise. Then, during your next workout, attempt to do more. When you are comfortably lifting between twelve and sixteen repetitions, increase the amount of training weight for your next exercise session.

Weeks 1 and 2: Choose: 1 exercise for your back
Perform one set of each 1 exercise for your chest
1 exercise for your shoulders
1 exercise for your biceps
1 exercise for your triceps
1 exercise for your quadriceps
1 exercise for your hamstrings
Beginning abdominals

Weeks 3 and 4: Choose: 2 exercises for your back
Perform one set of each 2 exercises for your chest
1 exercise for your shoulders
1 exercise for your biceps
1 exercise for your triceps
1 exercise for your quadriceps
1 exercise for your hamstrings

---

1 exercise for your
calves
Abdominals

Weeks 5 and 6: Choose: 3 exercises for your back
Perform one set of each 2 exercises for your chest
2 exercises for your
shoulders
1 exercise for your
biceps
1 exercise for your
triceps
1 exercise for your
quadriceps
1 exercise for your
hamstrings
1 exercise for your total
legs/buttocks
1 exercise for your
calves
Abdominals

Weeks 7 and 8: Begin two sets of each exercise.
Continue adding variety to your
program.

Maintenance: Continue at two to three sets of
each exercise.
Mix up your workout, allowing for
variety.
Continue to increase weight when
needed.

GUIDELINES:
- Complete this routine 2 or 3 times a week (a minimum of twice).
- For upper body exercises stay within 10 to 15 repetition scheme. This means choosing a weight that will allow you to do at least 10 reps. Then, when you work your way up to 15 repetitions, add weight.
- For lower body exercises (your squats and lunges) stay between 15 and 20 reps. For your lunges that would mean 15 to 20 on each side.
- For your two body weight exercises (your push-ups and chair dips) go till you can't do anymore.

Weeks 1 and 2: do one set per exercise

Weeks 3 and 4: do two sets per exericise

Weeks 5 and 6: do three sets per exercise

Basic Strength Training

The following program is a basic routine that works all your major muscle groups. It is a good beginner's routine. The goal is to build a solid foundation so you can go to the next level. The routine was designed using minimal equipment (all you need is a set of dumbbells), so you can do it at home or the gym. It is important to perform the exercises in the order given.

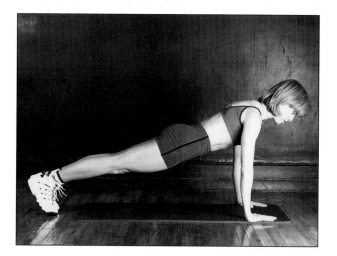

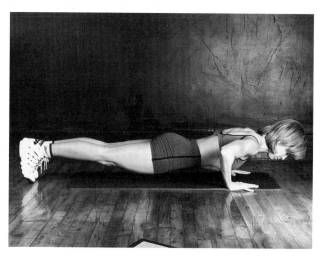

The Routine—Chest

EXERCISE: PUSH-UPS

STARTING POSITION: Lie on your stomach, elbows bent, palms facing down, placed on outside and even with your shoulders. Extend your legs straight back, toes tucked under your feet. Straighten your arms, lifting your entire body off the floor, balancing on your hands and the underside of your toes. Tighten your abdominal muscles to stabilize your body, while keeping your entire body aligned.

THE MOVEMENT: Bend your arms and lower your body until it makes contact with the floor, then straighten your arms, raising your torso back to the starting position (do not fully lock your elbows). This constitutes one repetition.

VARIATION: This exercise can also be done from your knees. Bend your knees so your lower legs are up in the air and you're balancing on your hands and knees.

TRAINER'S TIPS:
- Think of your body as a solid unit, moving as a whole.
- Keep your head and neck in alignment: don't look up or down.
- Concentrate on your chest as you go through the entire range of motion.
- Exhale as you push up, inhale as you go down.

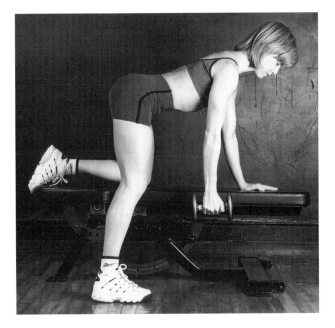
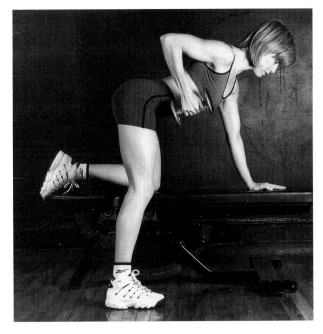

Back

EXERCISE: BENT ROW

STARTING POSITION: Place one hand on a bench for support (if you're using your right arm for lifting, use your left knee and hand for support). Then bend forward from your waist, creating about a 45-degree angle with your upper body, and tighten your ABs for stability. Grasp a dumbbell with your right hand, letting your arm hang straight down (palm facing in).

THE MOVEMENT: Using your back muscles, bend your right arm and pull the weight to your chest. Then lower in a controlled motion. Do the same number of repetitions with the other arm.

TRAINER'S TIPS:
- Imagine you have a string on your elbow and the movement is initiated from there, instead of the hand.
- Focus on pulling with your back muscles.
- Control the motion on both phases of the movement, don't let gravity take over.
- Exhale as you pull the weight toward your chest. Inhale as you lower the weight.

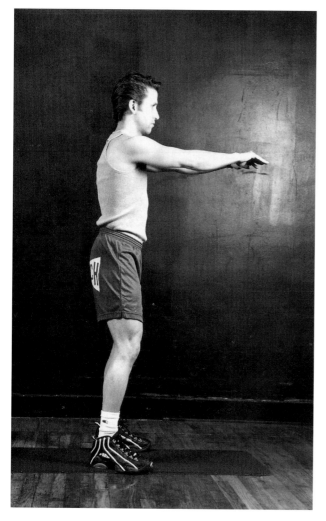

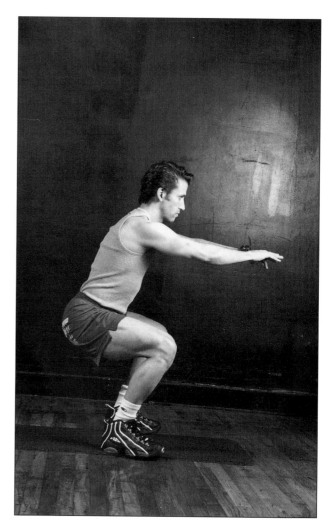

Legs

EXERCISE: THE SQUAT

STARTING POSITION: Prepare to squat by first setting your lower body: feet comfortably apart (shoulder width in most cases), toes pointed slightly out, knees slightly bent, and weight distributed from the balls of your feet to your heels. Next, set your upper body: chest out, shoulders back, lower back neither arched nor rounded, head in alignment with your spine, eyes looking straight ahead.

THE MOVEMENT: Descend in a controlled manner (your hips moving backward as if you're sitting and your torso leaning forward) until the tops of your thighs are parallel to the ground. Don't let your knees come out over your toes. Return to starting position.

TRAINER'S TIPS:
- You can add weight by holding dumbbells at your sides.
- Don't bounce at the bottom of the movement.
- Keep heels flat.
- Don't allow your hips to sway backward as you come up.
- Focus your mind on your thigh muscles.

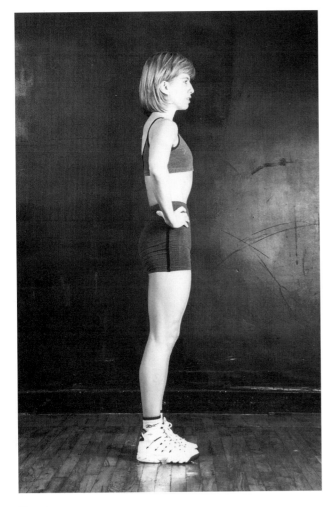 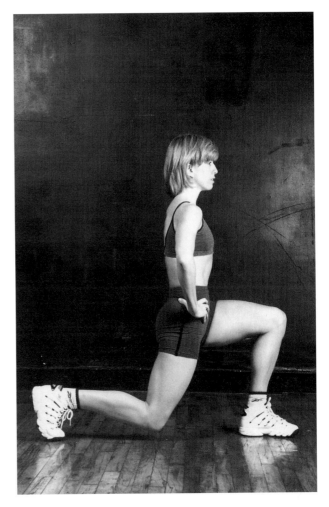

Legs

EXERCISE: LUNGES

STARTING POSITION: Prepare to lunge by first setting your lower body: feet shoulder-width apart, toes pointed straight ahead, knees slightly bent, and weight distributed evenly on your feet. Next, set your upper body: chest out, shoulders back, lower back neither arched nor rounded, head in alignment with your spine, eyes looking straight ahead.

THE MOVEMENT: Step forward with either leg, a little longer than your normal stride length, landing heel to toe. Stop just short of letting your back knee touch the ground. Do not let the knee of your front leg drive over your toe. Push back with your front leg to return to starting position. Repeat with same leg or alternate legs.

TRAINER'S TIPS:
- You can add weight by holding dumbbells at your sides.
- Keep your back and neck aligned.
- Make sure your hips drop straight down, not forward.
- Don't bounce your knee off the ground.
- Your eyes should look straight ahead throughout movement.

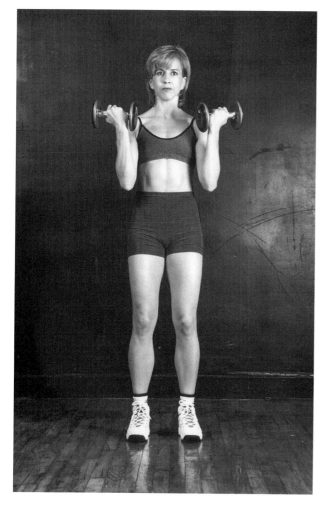
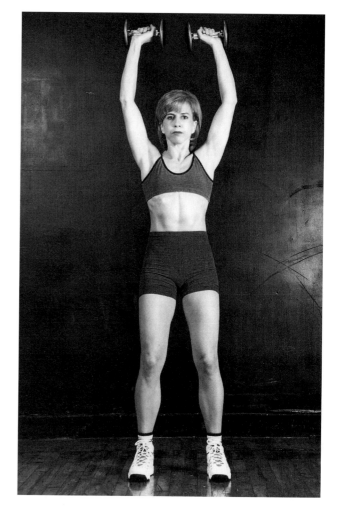

Shoulders

EXERCISE: ROTATION PRESS

STARTING POSITION: Sit on edge of bench or stand with feet shoulder-width apart and knees slightly bent. Hold both dumbbells underneath your chin with your hands rotated so that the back of your hands face forward. Your chest should be up, with both shoulders pulled slightly back and your eyes looking straight ahead.

THE MOVEMENT: As you raise both dumbbells directly over your head, rotate both hands so that your palms face forward when your arms are fully extended over your head. Bring both dumbbells together at the top as you straighten your arms. Return to starting position under control.

TRAINER'S TIPS:
- Maintain good posture throughout exercise.
- Avoid arching your lower back as you lift.
- Focus your mind on your shoulders throughout the exercise.

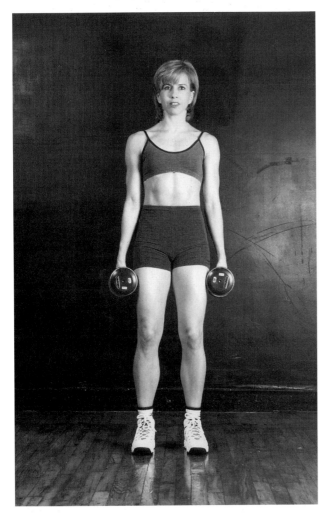 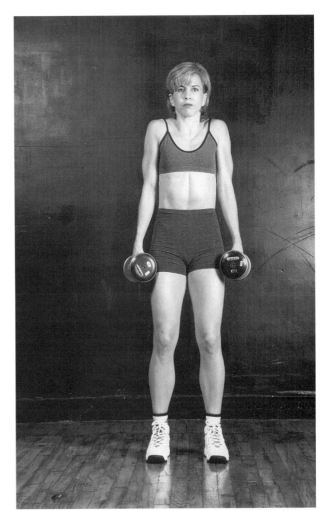

Trapezius

EXERCISE: SHRUGS

STARTING POSITION: Stand (knees slightly bent) holding two dumbbells at your sides (palms facing in).

THE MOVEMENT: Keeping proper back alignment (back straight, chest out, eyes straight ahead), elevate dumbbells by raising your shoulders toward your ears. Once the shoulders are elevated completely, drop chin (this should raise your shoulders higher) and hold for a count. Return to starting position in a controlled manner. Repeat for the prescribed number of repetitions.

TRAINER'S TIPS:
- Make sure to squeeze at the top of the contraction.
- Keep good postural alignment.
- Don't lean back.
- Don't come up on your toes.

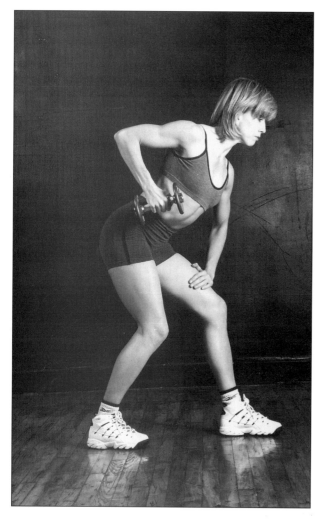

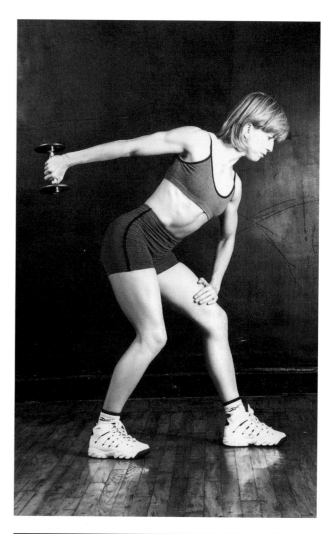

Triceps

EXERCISE: DUMBBELL KICKBACKS

STARTING POSITION: Rest your left knee on a bench, bend forward, placing your left hand on the bench or your thigh for support. Holding a dumbbell, bend your arm at the elbow and elevate your elbow as high as possible. Avoid dipping your shoulder, and keep the upper arm perpendicular to the ground.

THE MOVEMENT: Keeping your upper arm pressed to your side with the elbow elevated, push the dumbbell up and out until your arm is fully extended. Return under control to original starting position.

TRAINER'S TIPS:
- Maintain good position throughout exercise.
- Keep the elbow elevated throughout the exercise.
- Focus your mind on your triceps.

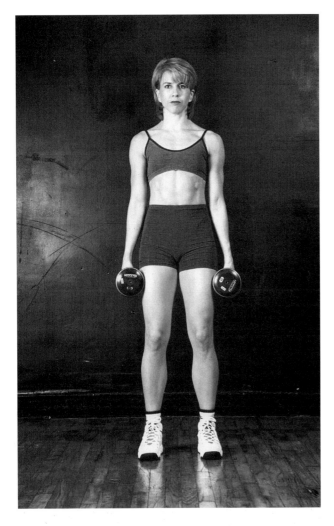
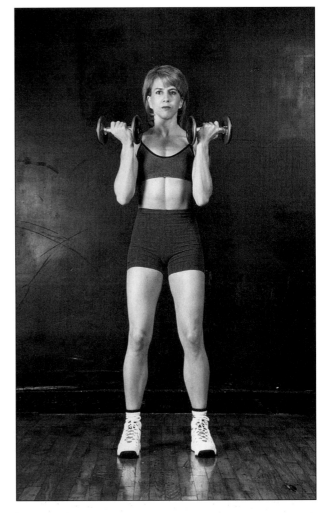

Biceps

EXERCISE: STANDING DUMBBELL CURLS

STARTING POSITION: Stand with feet shoulder-width apart, grasping two dumbbells with arms hanging straight at your sides, palms facing in.

THE MOVEMENT: As you begin the curl movement with both dumbbells simultaneously, rotate your palms up and continue to curl in a smooth arc to your shoulder. Then lower the dumbbells back to the starting position.

TRAINER'S TIPS:
- Keep your upper arms motionless and pressed against your upper torso throughout range of movement.
- Aim for a smooth, flowing movement.
- Do not allow a sudden drop or drag on shoulder socket at bottom of movement.
- You may stand with back flat against the wall for added back support.
- Focus your mind on working muscles.

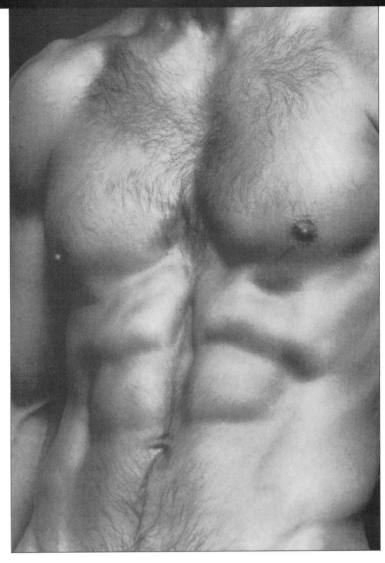

The Exercises

**APPROXIMATELY HOW MANY CALORIES DOES
TWENTY CRUNCHES BURN OFF?**

Nine

Introduction to the Exercises

There are hundreds of exercises and variations for your ABs. Most exercise books give you only ten or so to choose from. In the next five chapters, you will learn over a hundred. The purpose of this extensive selection is to offer you a wide variety of exercises, so you can find those that work best for you. Also, variety reduces boredom and promotes continued adaptation.

The Groupings

The exercises are grouped in the areas they emphasize: Area One (Lower ABs), Area Two (Obliques), Area Three (Upper ABs), Area Four (Combination—works two or more areas), and Isometric exercises. Similar exercises are grouped together when possible. For example, Crunches, Sit-ups, Hanging Leg Move-

ments are put in groups. These groupings make it easier to see variations in the exercises.

Usage Guidelines

Each exercise has guidelines to help you make intelligent choices. The following section explains these guidelines.

DIFFICULTY LEVELS The exercises are ranked from 1 to 3: 1 being the easiest, 2, intermediate, and 3, advanced. Choose exercises that correspond to your fitness level and exercise experience. These, of course, are general categories. Depending on your individual strengths and weaknesses, you will find particular exercises more or less difficult than the next person. Remember, increasing difficulty is a way to increase intensity and cause muscle adaptation. So start with the easier exercises, build strength, and move to more difficult movements.

LOWER BACK Everybody's lower back is different. The purpose of these rankings is not to discourage you from doing certain exercises or encourage you to do those that will prove too strenuous. They are a warning to proceed carefully. If you have a history of lower-back problems, you need to exercise with extra care. You should also consult a doctor to discuss exercise in relation to your specific problem. Again, these rankings are general guidelines to help you find the appropriate exercises that fit your needs and experience.

The three lower-back rankings are: Low Risk, Moderate Risk, High Risk. These rankings are based on a combination of the following criteria:

1. *The range of motion involved in the movement.* Smaller, isolated movements such as a crunch are safer than a full sit-up.
2. *Single or compound plane of movement.* A single plane of movement is safer than a compound movement. For example, a straight crunch takes place on a single plane, as opposed to a crunch with a twist, which takes place on two planes: up and down and rotation. Single-plane movements are generally safer.
3. *Single or compound movement.* A single movement would involve either the leg or the torso working alone, as in a crunch or a side leg raise. A compound movement involves two areas working together, as in a jackknife. Single-plane movements are generally safer.
4. *Length of the lever involved in the movement.* The longer the lever (torso or legs) is and the farther away it moves from your center in its range of motion, the more torque (stress) on the lower back. Therefore, straight leg movements and full sit-ups place more stress on the lower back than crunch or bent-leg movements.
5. *External support.* The more external support the lower back has, the safer the movement will be. So,

any movement where you keep your lower back against the floor is generally safer than movement without such support.

These criteria are not carved in stone. There will be exceptions to the rules. But knowing these general principles gives you the tools to modify certain exercises to fit your lower-back needs.

AREA This section gives the name of the muscle or muscles you are working. Being able to correctly visualize the area you are working is an essential element for visualization.

INSTRUCTION Here is the exercise itself, starting position, movement, proper exercise technique.

TRAINER'S TIPS This section acts as your personal trainer. Some of the tips will be specific to the exercise. Others will be constant reminders, tips that are true for every exercise. You need to hear these tips over and over until they become second nature. The following tips are essential for AB work:

• Keep constant tension on the ABs.
• Keep motion slow and controlled, no bouncing or jerking.
• Hold total contraction at the top of the movement.
• Don't rest at the bottom of the movement before starting your next repetition.
• When possible, keep lower back supported.
• Focus your mind on feeling your ABs do the work.

SPEED OF MOVEMENT An important element of variety is the speed of movement during an exercise. General speed guidelines are:

Fast: About one rep every second
Medium: About one rep every two seconds
Slow: About one rep every five seconds

This element becomes more important as your training becomes more advanced. You can do exercises within a routine at different speeds or break up your routines with a slow day, fast day, and medium-speed day.

PULSING Pulsing is holding a movement at the top of its range of motion, then moving back and forth, about one to two inches, keeping constant tension on the ABs. This tiny movement pumps the muscle. The effect is like making a loose fist, squeeze it tight, let it slightly relax, squeeze it tight, and let it slightly relax.

EXERCISE VARIETY Similar exercises are grouped together in a series. These exercises have similar movements with different variations added: for example, the crunch series. In each exercise, you do the same crunch movement, but there are a variety of leg positions. Although the movements are similar, the different leg positions hit the muscle from slightly different angles. The more angles you hit the muscle from, the better overall strength and aesthetics you will achieve.

Using the different leg position is key in achieving one of the important training principles—variety. Without variety you will get bored, the muscle will grow complacent, instead of being shocked into growth periods.

CONTROVERSIAL EXERCISES Other exercises in this section that may be considered by some dangerous and ineffective, because they don't isolate the ABs. They either involve other muscles, such as the hip flexors and lower back, or their range of motion goes past the effective limit to isolate the ABs.

There is truth in this. All of the straight-leg movements and full sit-ups will involve the hip flexors and other secondary muscles to complete the movement. But the principles of variety and shocking the muscle with new exercises from new angles also hold true for these movements. And certain sport-specific routines use these exercises because the chain of muscles they train are specific to the movements in many sports. Some exercise physiologists are changing their minds about the virtues of straight sit-ups. One of the goals of this book is to give both points of view on controversial issues surrounding the ABs.

These exercises are, of course, difficult, and shouldn't be used by those with lower-back problems, the elderly, or those just starting out.

Hand Positions

Hand position is an important part of each exercise. When you're working your ABs, there are three basic hand positions.

HANDS EXTENDED This position shifts the resistance forward, decreasing the work load. This is a good position for beginners and those having difficulty doing the recommended number of reps.

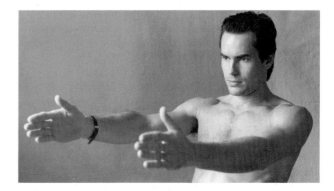

HANDS ACROSS CHEST This is an intermediate position where the weight is shifted back, increasing the work load.

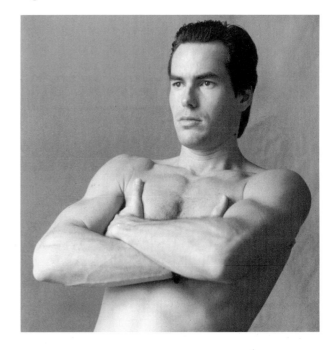

ONE HAND VARIATION The following variation is also a position of choice. It can help reduce neck strain. Neck strain originates from holding the weight of your head up. To counter this problem, you can hold the weight of your head in one of your hands. The key is to let the weight rest in the hand, placing the stress on the arm and shoulder and taking it off your neck. Then place your free hand on the area of the abdomen you are working (upper, sides, or lower ABs). Feeling the muscle work will help focus your mind and inspire you to do a couple more reps.

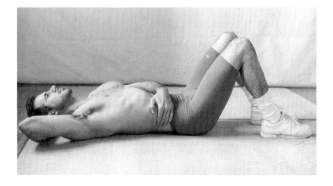

HANDS BEHIND EARS: This position shifts the weight back and up, giving the most resistance. **You should *not* interlock your fingers and pull your head forward, as you may have been taught in P.E. class.** You should have your fingers and hands supporting your head. Experiment with these different positions. On some exercises, the resistance with the different hand positions may seem substantial; in others it may seem insignificant. And some exercises can be executed only using a particular hand position.

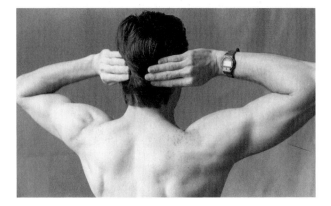

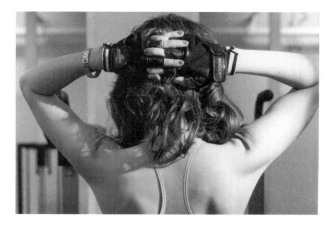

HEAD POSITION. When doing AB work you should always try to maintain a fist's distance between your chin and chest.

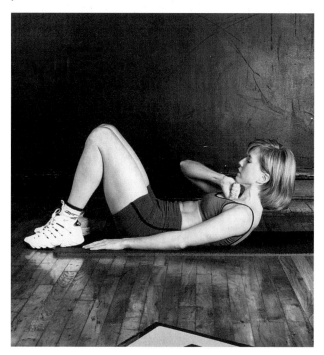

Weight Resistance

You can add weight resistance on almost any AB exercise. This is normally done with the use of weight plates, dumbbells, or a medicine ball. Adding weight to an exercise will increase intensity. The safest way to add weight is to place the weights across your chest. The safest way to add weight for leg movements is to hold a dumbbell between your feet. When adding resistance, you may find a medicine ball the most comfortable. The best way to hold it is to simply place it between your knees and gently squeeze. Other alternatives are holding weight behind your head. Or, for some exercises, you will need to hold weight extended in front of your body.

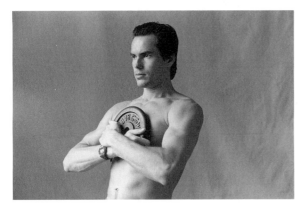

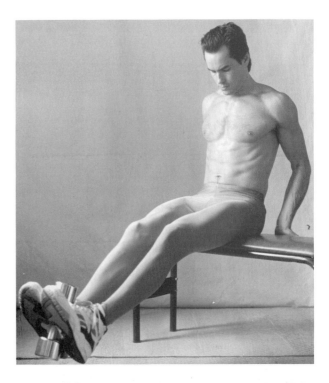

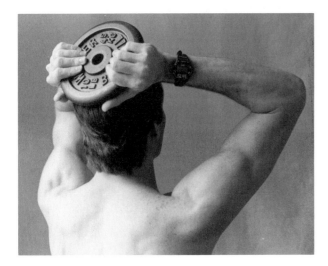

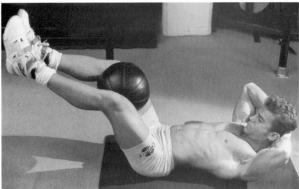

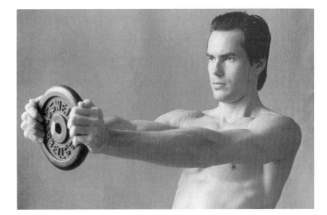

Adding weights to an AB routine is an advanced technique—for serious bodybuilders and athletes only. Using weights will add mass (size) to your abdomen, a look many people don't want. In general, you should start by using the lightest weights available (one to three pounds) and add weight very slowly, in small increments. Because of the risk of injury, heavy weights are not recommended for AB training. Never use so much weight that you can't finish your target number of reps. The most important thing is not to recruit other muscle groups besides your ABs to complete the exercise. A breakdown in proper technique defeats the purpose of the exercise and increases your risk of injury. The rule for weight training in general applies here: You have to give yourself at least one day's rest between using weights.

STARTING POSITION FOR LEG RAISES

Some of these exercises involve lying on your back on the floor and raising your legs. This position warrants a special discussion because correct position can help prevent lower-back problems. Everybody is different, so finding the best position may involve some trial and error. Placing the hands, palms down, under the bottom part of your buttocks, with your elbows at your sides, shoulder blades just off the floor, and chin to your chest, is an effective way to keep your lower back pressed against the floor. Placing your hands at the bottom of your buttocks instead of directly under them allows your hands to act as a wedge, pushing your hips up and into a pelvic tilt. This slight hip elevation will keep your back pressed against the floor, helping to protect you throughout the two most dangerous points of the movement: the beginning and the end.

On all starting positions, do what is most comfortable and feels the least dangerous to you, without destroying the integrity of the exercise. If you need a pillow or towel under your head, neck, lower back, buttocks, or knees, put one there. Comfort and safety should come first.

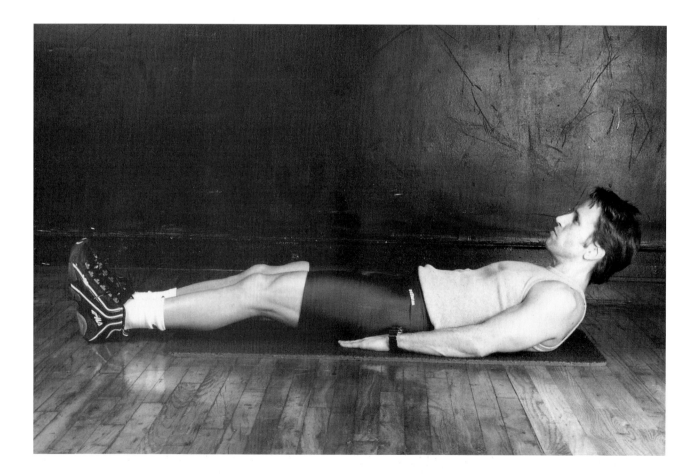

CHAPTER TEN

Area One: The Lower ABs

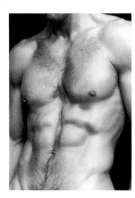

Exercise: Reverse Crunches

DIFFICULTY: 1
LOWER BACK: LOW RISK
AREA: LOWER ABS

STARTING POSITION: Lie flat on your back with your head up (chin to chest). Your legs are up so your thighs are perpendicular to your body, placing your calves and feet parallel to the floor. Have your hands at your sides, or lightly placed at the sides of the head.

MOVEMENT: Use your lower ABs to raise your hips off the floor toward your rib cage, arching your knees toward your forehead. Lower your hips in a controlled motion, keeping tension on your ABs. When your hips make light contact with the floor, pull the knees back up toward your forehead. Repeat.

TRAINER'S TIPS:
- Make sure the lower ABs are doing the work. Don't rock, using momentum.
- Don't rest your hips on the floor at the bottom of the movement.
- Keep constant tension on the ABs.
- Focus your mind on feeling your ABs do the work.
- Use your hands for balance. Don't use them to push off.

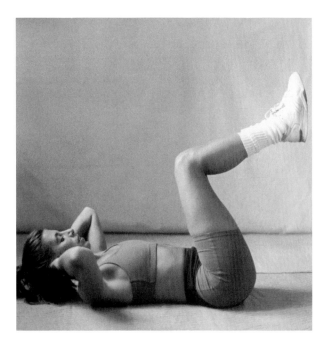
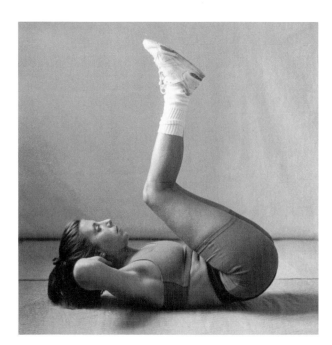

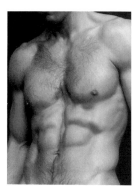

Exercise: Bench Reverse Crunches

DIFFICULTY: 2
LOWER BACK: MODERATE RISK
AREA: LOWER ABS

STARTING POSITION: Lie on your back on a bench, positioning your legs up so your thighs are perpendicular to your body and your lower legs are parallel to the floor. Then let your hips slide off the edge of the bench.

MOVEMENT: Use your lower ABs to curl your hips up and over the bench toward your rib cage. Then lower your hips below the bench and repeat.

TRAINER'S TIPS:
- Keep constant tension on your lower ABs throughout the full range of motion (both raising and lowering).
- Make sure you lower your hips below the bench on each repetition.
- Raise the hips as high as you would on a normal reverse crunch.
- Don't rest at the bottom of the movement.
- Focus your mind on your lower ABs.

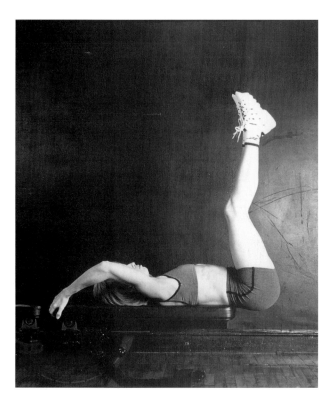

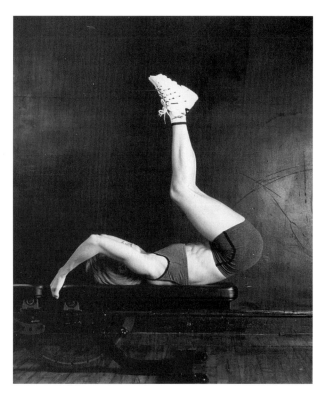

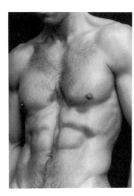

Exercise: Hip Raises

DIFFICULTY: 3
LOWER BACK: MODERATE RISK
AREA: LOWER ABS

STARTING POSITION: Lie flat on your back with your legs extended straight up (knees unlocked). Place your hands at your sides, palms down, and bring your chin toward your chest.

MOVEMENT: Use your lower ABs to elevate your hips off the floor, shifting your weight toward your shoulders. Then lower yourself back down in a controlled motion until your hips make light contact with the floor. Repeat.

TRAINER'S TIPS:
- Don't kick with the legs to help elevate the hips—make the ABs do the work.
- Use your hands to help maintain balance, and not to help push your hips up.
- Hold total contraction at the top of the movement for a count of two.
- Focus your mind on feeling your ABs do the work.

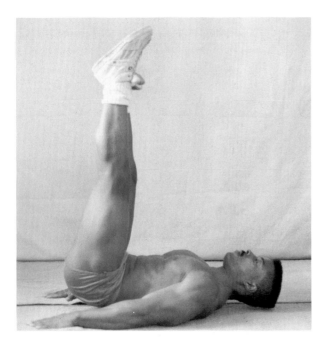

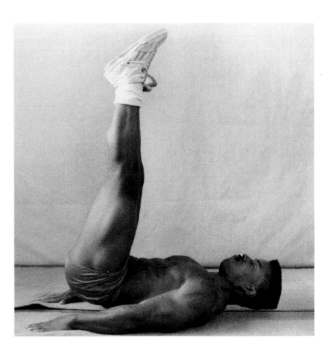

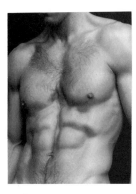

Exercise: Bench Hip Raises

DIFFICULTY: 3
LOWER BACK: MODERATE RISK
AREA: LOWER ABS

STARTING POSITION: Lie on your back on a bench with your legs extended straight up (knees unlocked), and grab the sides of the bench to stabilize your body. Then slide your hips off the edge of the bench.

MOVEMENT: Use your lower ABs to elevate your hips straight up. Then lower your hips below the bench and repeat.

TRAINER'S TIPS:
- Raise the hips as high as you would on a normal hip raise.
- Keep constant tension on your lower ABs throughout the full range of motion (both raising and lowering).
- Make sure you lower your hips below bench on each repetition.
- Don't rest at the bottom of the movement.
- Focus your mind on your lower ABs.

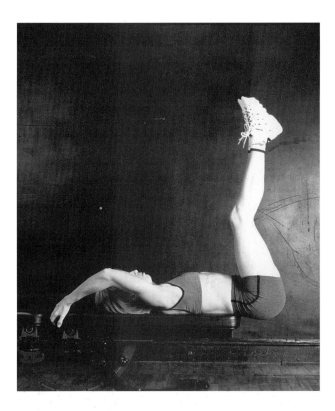

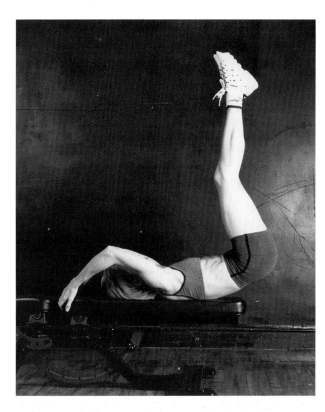

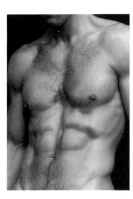

Exercise: Bent-Leg Hip Raises

DIFFICULTY: 2
LOWER BACK: LOW RISK
AREA: LOWER ABS

STARTING POSITION: Lie on the floor, knees bent, heels on the floor, and your head up (chin toward chest). Hands in position of choice.

MOVEMENT: Keeping the feet together, use your lower ABs to raise your hips off the floor, bringing your knees toward your forehead. At the top of the movement, your feet should be over your head. Then lower your legs back down, letting your feet lightly touch the floor. Repeat.

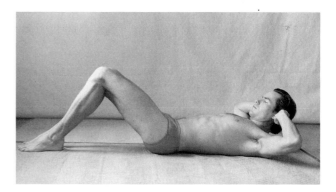

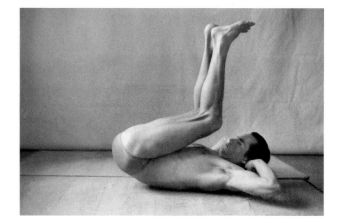

TRAINER'S TIPS:
- Don't swing your legs back, using momentum to help get your hips off the floor.
- Don't let the legs drop on the way down. Lower them slowly, keeping tension on the ABs.
- Hold a total contraction at the top of the movement for a count of two.
- Focus your mind on feeling your lower ABs do the work.

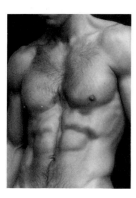

Exercise: Knee Raises

DIFFICULTY: 2
LOWER BACK: LOW RISK
AREA: LOWER ABS

STARTING POSITION: Lie on the floor (on your back), hands under your buttocks (palms down), elbows out so the small of your back is pressed against the floor, head up (chin to chest), shoulder blades off the floor. Then extend your legs straight out (knees unlocked), heels resting on the floor.

MOVEMENT: Use the muscles of your lower ABs to draw your knees up to your chest. Then lower in a controlled motion, keeping a slight bend in the knees. Let the heels lightly brush the floor. Repeat.

Variation: This same movement can be done on an incline board.

TRAINER'S TIPS:
- Keep your lower back pressed against the floor or incline board.
- Hold a total contraction at the top of the movement for a count of two.
- Focus your mind on feeling the lower ABs do the work.

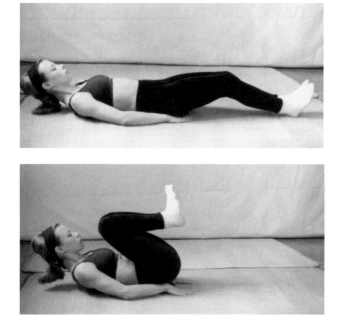

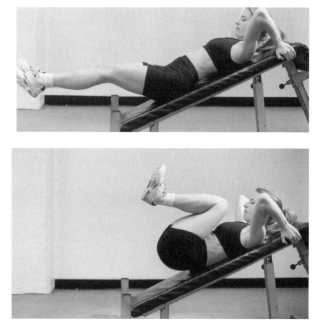

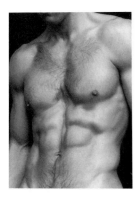

Exercise: Knee Raises: Cycling

DIFFICULTY: 2
LOWER BACK: MODERATE RISK
AREA: LOWER ABS

STARTING POSITION: Lie on the floor (on your back), hands under your buttocks (palms down), elbows out so the small of your back is pressed against the floor, head up (chin to chest), shoulder blades off the floor. Then extend your legs straight out (knees unlocked), heels resting on the floor.

MOVEMENT. Lift both legs approximately one foot off the floor, with a slight bend in the knees. Use your lower ABs to draw your right knee to your chest. Extend the leg out as you simultaneously draw the left leg toward your chest. The two legs should cross at the midpoint of the movement. Each time both legs have been raised toward the shoulders equals one repetition. The motion is similar to pedaling a bike.

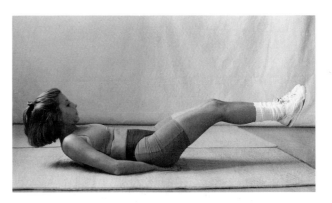

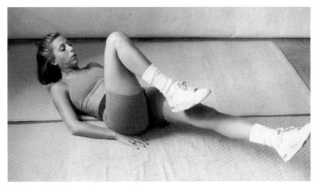

TRAINER'S TIPS:
- Make sure not to let either foot touch the floor—keep constant tension on the ABs.
- Keep motion controlled. Don't go too fast.
- Feel the legs being pulled and extended by the AB muscles, not the leg and hip flexors.
- Focus your mind on feeling your lower ABs do the work.
- If you have lower-back problems, raising the legs higher than a foot off the floor will relieve pressure.

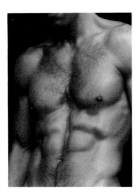

Exercise: Modified Knee Raises

DIFFICULTY: 1
LOWER BACK: LOW RISK
AREA: LOWER ABS

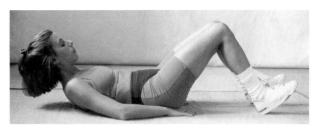

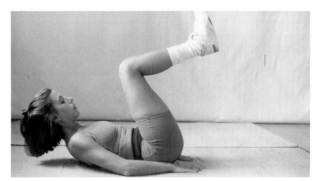

STARTING POSITION: Lie on the floor (on your back), hands under your buttocks (palms down), elbows out so the small of your back is pressed against the floor, head up (chin to chest), shoulder blades off the floor. Then bend your knees, resting your feet flat on the floor.

MOVEMENT: From this modified position, use your lower ABs to draw your knees to your chest. Then lower your legs until your heels lightly touch the floor. Repeat.

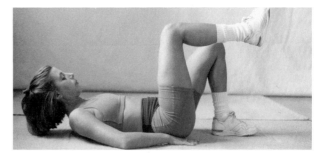

Single-Leg Variation: Execute the same movement, from the same starting position, but raise only one leg at a time. Complete one side, then switch legs.

Single-Leg Variation: One Leg Up —Raise one leg so your thigh is perpendicular with your torso and your foot is parallel to the floor. Your other leg is bent, with your foot flat on the floor. Raise the bent knee, bringing it toward your chest, and lower it, letting your heel lightly touch the ground. Repeat. Then switch sides. The opposite leg stays up throughout the exercise.

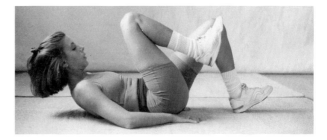

TRAINER'S TIPS:
- Concentrate on just bringing knees to the chest and touching heels to the ground.
- Don't worry about getting the hips off the floor— they will raise a little naturally when you bring the knees to the chest.
- Hold a total contraction at the top of the movement for a count of two.
- Don't let your feet rest at the bottom of the movement.
- This is a good exercise for beginners.

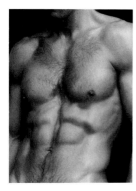

Exercise: Seated Knee Raises

DIFFICULTY: 2
LOWER BACK: LOW RISK
AREA: LOWER ABS

STARTING POSITION: Sit on the edge of a bench or chair holding on to the back or side of the bench for support, legs extended, heels just off the floor, and upper body upright.

MOVEMENT: Use the muscles of your lower ABs to draw your knees toward your chest. Then lower in a controlled motion, keeping a slight bend in the knees. Let the heels lightly brush the floor, then repeat the movement. Keep your upper body stationary during the movement, simply pulling the knees up to the chest.

TRAINER'S TIPS:
- Control the motion on the way down, keeping tension on the ABs.
- Focus your mind on feeling your lower ABs do the work.
- Hold a total contraction at the top of the movement for a count of two.
- Be careful not to lean your torso too far back. Keep it upright.

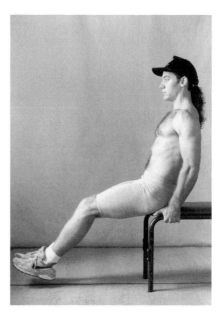

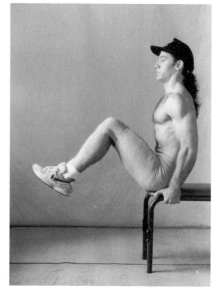

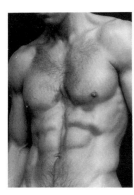

Exercise: Leg Raises

DIFFICULTY: 2
LOWER BACK: HIGH RISK
AREA: LOWER ABS

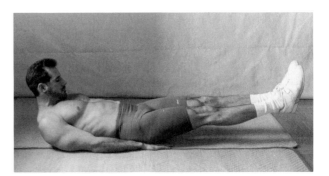

STARTING POSITION: Lie on the floor (on your back), hands under your buttocks (palms down), elbows out so the small of your back is pressed against the floor, head up (chin to chest), shoulder blades off the floor. Then extend your legs straight out (knees unlocked), heels resting on the floor.

MOVEMENT: Use the muscles of your lower ABs to raise your legs until they are perpendicular to the body. Then lower the legs in a controlled motion. Repeat.

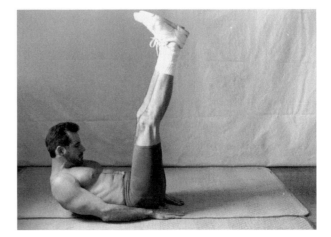

Variation: This movement can also be done on an incline board and/or as a single-leg exercise.

TRAINER'S TIPS:
- Keep your lower back pressed against the floor.
- Keep a slight bend in your knees at all times.
- At the top of the movement, hold a total contraction for a count of two.
- Don't rest your feet on the floor at the bottom of the movement.
- Focus your mind on feeling your lower ABs do the work.

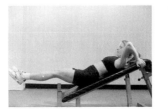

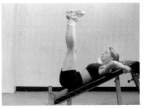

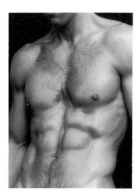

Exercise: Leg Raises: Alternating

DIFFICULTY: 2
LOWER BACK: HIGH RISK
AREA: LOWER ABS

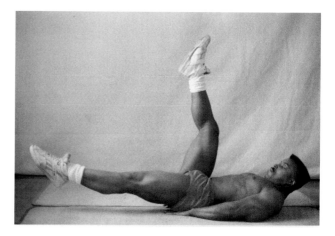

STARTING POSITION: Lie on the floor (on your back), hands under your buttocks (palms down), elbows out so the small of your back is pressed against the floor, head up (chin to chest), shoulder blades off the floor. Then extend your legs straight out (knees unlocked), heels resting on the floor.

MOVEMENT: Using the muscles of your lower ABs, raise your right leg (with a slight bend at the knee) until it is perpendicular with your body (a 90-degree angle). Then, in a controlled motion, lower it back to the floor. As you start to lower it, raise your left leg to the perpendicular position. They should pass each other midway. One repetition is completed when both legs have gone to the raised position.

MOVEMENT VARIATION: Bring one leg up, lower it, then raise the other leg up and lower it, instead of keeping constant motion. This variation is less stressful on the lower back.

TRAINER'S TIPS:
- Keep your lower back pressed against the floor.
- Focus your mind on feeling your lower ABs do the work.
- Don't let either leg rest on the floor at the bottom of the movement.
- Keep the motion controlled.

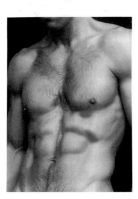

Exercise: Leg Raises with Movement Sequences

DIFFICULTY: 3
LOWER BACK: HIGH RISK
AREA: LOWER ABS

STARTING POSITION: Lie on the floor (on your back), hands under your buttocks (palms down), elbows out so the small of your back is pressed against the floor, head up (chin to chest), shoulder blades off the floor. Then extend your legs straight out (knees unlocked), heels resting on the floor.

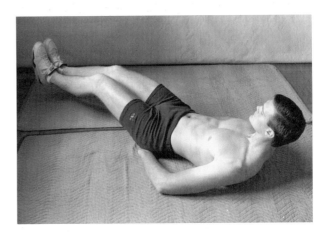

MOVEMENT: Raise legs approximately one foot off the floor with a slight bend in the knees and hold position. Move the legs in the following motions:

Figure Eights. Raise your legs slightly above a 45-degree angle, and on the wall in front of you draw an imaginary figure eight with your feet down to the starting position and back up. Switch directions after each figure is drawn. Continue until you complete your set.

Circles: Draw circles with your feet, switch directions with the completion of each circle. Continue movement until you complete your set.

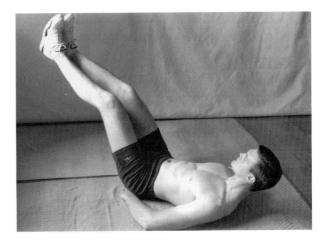

Crisscrosses: From the starting position, crisscross your legs back and forth, alternating top and bottom positions with your legs. Each cross counts as a rep.

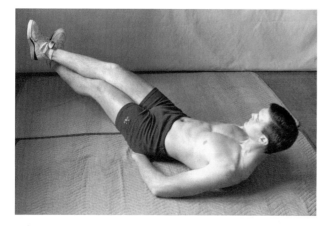

Kicks: From the starting position, you will move your legs up and down. To start the exercise, raise right leg about a foot above the left leg. Then reverse position, raising the left leg and lowering the right leg. Continue this motion until you complete your set. Each time a leg changes positions counts as a repetition.

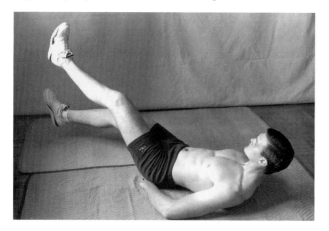

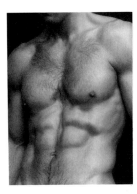

Exercise: Hanging Knee Raises

DIFFICULTY: 2
LOWER BACK: LOW RISK
AREA: LOWER ABS

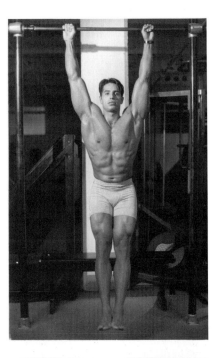

STARTING POSITION: Hang from a bar or vertical chair, legs fully extended.

MOVEMENT: Use the muscles of your lower ABs to raise the knees to the chest, letting the hips move forward as the knees pass the 90-degree angle. Your feet should hang down below your knees. Then lower them in a controlled motion back to the starting position. Repeat.

TRAINER'S TIPS:
- Bring the knees as high up on the chest as possible.
- At the top of the movement, hold a full contraction for a count of two.
- When your legs are fully extended at the bottom of the movement, don't rest down there—bring the legs right back up for the next repetition.
- This is a good movement to build strength for Straight-Leg Hanging Raises.
- If you have problems getting the knees up to the chest, don't worry: Your range of motion will improve with work.
- Focus your mind on feeling your lower ABs do the work.

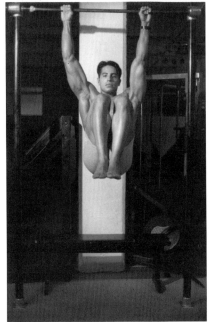

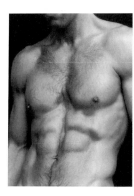

Exercise: Hanging Knee Raises: Alternating

DIFFICULTY: 2
LOWER BACK: LOW RISK
AREA: LOWER ABS

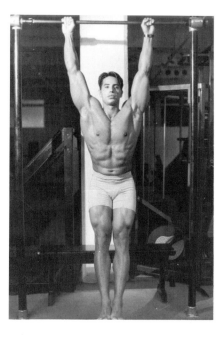

STARTING POSITION: Hang from a bar or vertical chair, legs fully extended.

MOVEMENT: Using the muscles of your lower ABs, bring your right knee up to your chest, then lower it. Repeat the movement with your left leg. Alternate until you complete your set.

TRAINER'S TIPS:
- Bring the knees up as high on the chest as possible.
- At the top of the movement, hold a total contraction for a count of two.
- Let the hips come forward after the knees pass the 90-degree angle.
- Don't rest at the bottom of the movement—keep constant tension on the ABs.
- Focus your mind on feeling the lower ABs do the work.
- This exercise can be done by alternating the movement or by doing multiple repetitions on one side and then switching.

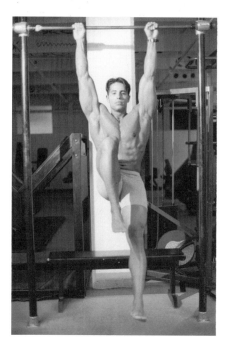

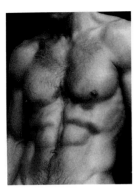

Exercise: Hanging Knee Raises: Bicycles

DIFFICULTY: 2
LOWER BACK: MODERATE RISK
AREA: LOWER ABS

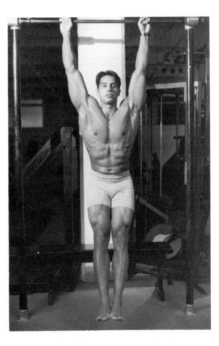

STARTING POSITION: Hang from a bar or vertical chair, legs fully extended.

MOVEMENT: Use the muscles of your lower ABs to move your legs as if you were pedaling a bicycle. Raise your right knee toward your chest; as you begin to lower it, simultaneously raise your left knee. The knees should pass each other at the midpoint of the movement. The left knee continues to the chest, and the right knee completes its downward range of motion. Repeat.

TRAINER'S TIPS:
- Bring the knee as high on the chest as possible.
- Let the hips naturally roll forward when the knee passes through the 90-degree angle.
- Try not to swing too much. Keep the motion controlled.
- Focus your mind on feeling your ABs do the work.

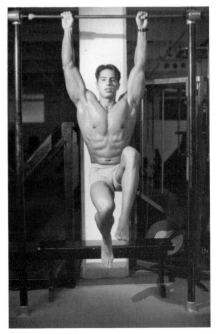

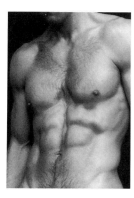

Exercise: Hanging Leg Raises: Straight Leg

DIFFICULTY: 3
LOWER BACK: HIGH RISK
AREA: LOWER ABS

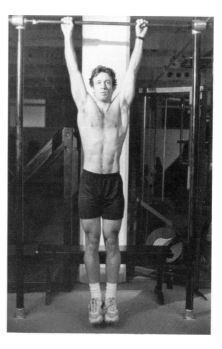

STARTING POSITION: Hang from a bar or vertical chair with your legs fully extended.

HALF LEG RAISES

MOVEMENT: Using the muscles of your lower ABs, raise your legs, keeping them straight (knees unlocked) until they are perpendicular with your upper body (90-degree angle). Then lower them in a controlled motion.

FULL LEG RAISES

MOVEMENT: Use the muscles of your lower ABs to raise your legs (knees unlocked) past the 90-degree angle until your feet are level with your chin.

TRAINER'S TIPS:
- Hold a total contraction at the top of the movement for a count of two.
- Lower the legs in a controlled motion. Don't just let them drop.
- Don't use a swinging motion to power your legs up.
- Focus your mind on feeling the lower AB muscles raising and lowering the legs.
- The Straight-Leg Raises activate the hip flexors more than the Bent-Leg Raises, but they are good for variety and for shocking the muscle.

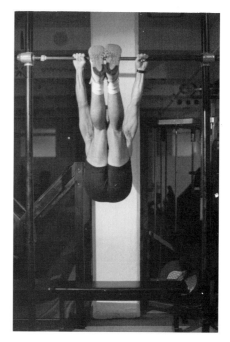

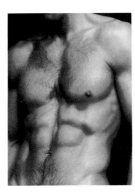

Exercise: Hanging Leg Raises: Bent Leg

DIFFICULTY: 3
LOWER BACK: MODERATE RISK
AREA: LOWER ABS

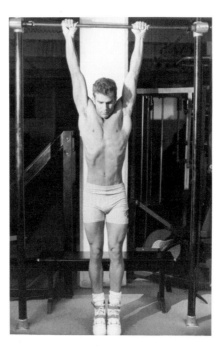

STARTING POSITION: Hang from a bar or a vertical chair, legs fully extended.

MOVEMENT: Use the muscles of your lower ABs to raise your legs, bringing your knees toward your forehead. At the top of the movement, your feet should be over your head. Then, in a controlled motion, lower them back to the starting position. Repeat.

TRAINER'S TIPS:
- Let your hips move forward as your legs curl toward your head.
- Try not to swing your legs to gain momentum.
- Control the motion on the way down.
- Hold a total contraction at the top of the movement for a count of two.
- Focus your mind on feeling your lower ABs do the work.

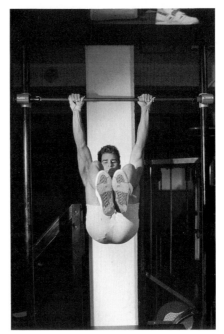

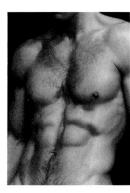

Exercise: Hanging Leg Raises: Alternating (Continuous Motion)

DIFFICULTY: 3
LOWER BACK: HIGH RISK
AREA: LOWER ABS

STARTING POSITION: Hang from a bar or vertical chair with your legs fully extended.

MOVEMENT: Use the muscles of your lower ABs to raise your right leg (knee joint unlocked) to about chin level. As you lower the right leg, simultaneously raise your left leg in the same manner. Your legs should cross each other going different directions at about the midpoint of the movement. The legs stay in continuous motion. Repeat the movement until you have completed your set.

TRAINER'S TIPS:
- Use the muscles of your lower ABs to raise and lower your legs.
- Let your hips come naturally out when your legs move past the 90-degree angle.
- Focus your mind on feeling the lower ABs do the work.
- Keep the movement controlled.
- If you can't get your feet to chin level, don't be discouraged: Your range of motion will increase with work.

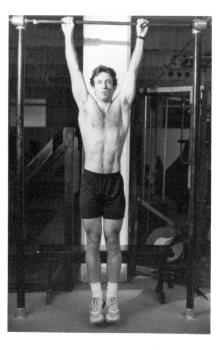

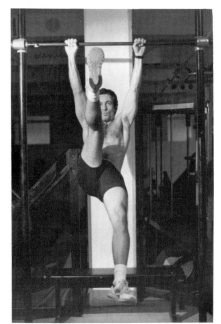

Exercise: Hanging Leg Raises:
Single Leg Straight

DIFFICULTY: 2
LOWER BACK: MODERATE RISK
AREA: LOWER ABS

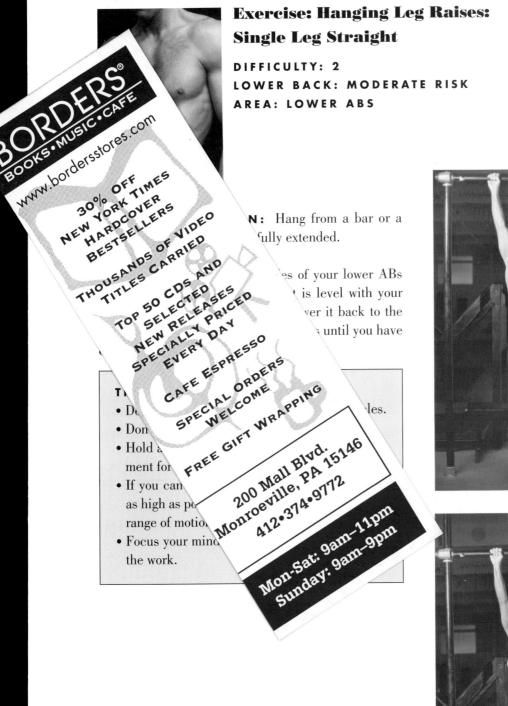

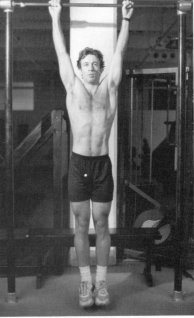

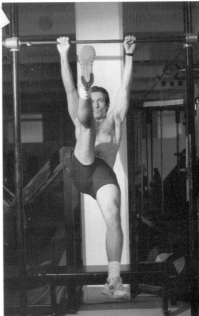

N : Hang from a bar or a
fully extended.

es of your lower ABs
t is level with your
ver it back to the
s until you have

T
• D   les.
• Don
• Hold a
  ment fo
• If you can
  as high as po
  range of motio
• Focus your min
  the work.

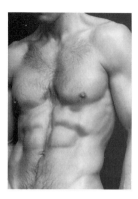

Exercise: Hanging Leg Raises with Movement Sequences

DIFFICULTY: 3
LOWER BACK: HIGH RISK
AREA: LOWER ABS

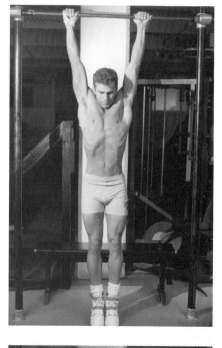

STARTING POSITION: Hang from a bar or vertical chair with your legs fully extended.

MOVEMENT: Use the muscles of your ABs to raise your legs to the L position (90-degree angle), keeping the knees unlocked. Then move the legs in the following motions:

Figure Eights: Raising your legs, draw an imaginary vertical eight with your feet on the wall in front of you. Switch directions after each figure eight. Repeat until you complete your set.

Circles: Raising your legs, draw imaginary circles with your feet on the wall in front of you. Switch directions with the completion of each circle. Continue movement until you complete your set.

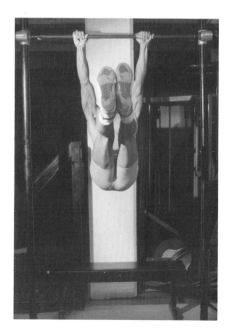

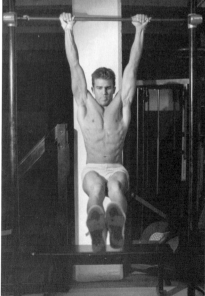

Crisscrosses: Move your legs horizontally, crisscrossing them back and forth. Your left leg moves to the right and crosses under the right leg. Then the motion reverses and your right leg crosses under the left and the left leg crosses above. Each time a leg crosses counts as a repetition.

Kicks: This time the legs move in a vertical motion. To start the exercise, raise the right leg about a foot and lower the left leg about a foot. Then reverse position, raise left leg and lower right leg, and reverse again. Each time a leg changes positions counts as a repetition.

TRAINER'S TIPS:
- Keep all motions controlled.
- Change the size and speed of your movements to add variety to your workout.
- Focus your mind on feeling your ABs do the work.

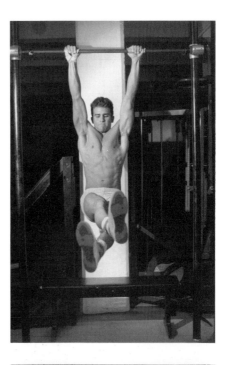

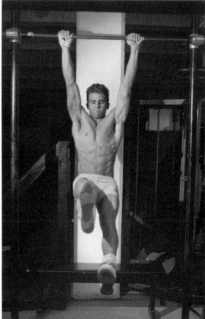

CHAPTER ELEVEN

Area Two: The Obliques

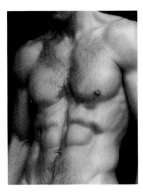

Exercise: Side Leg Raises

DIFFICULTY: 1
LOWER BACK: LOW RISK
AREA: OBLIQUES

STARTING POSITION: Lie on your side, resting on your left hip, left leg bent under your body, and rest on your tricep for support. From this position, extend your upper leg.

MOVEMENT: Use your oblique muscles to raise the upper leg as high as it will go without moving your hip, then lower it just short of the floor. Repeat the movement until you have completed your set. Then switch sides.

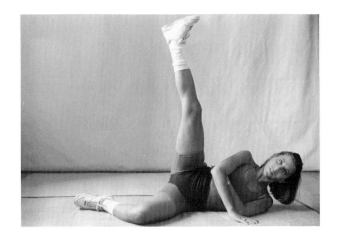

TRAINER'S TIPS:
- Don't swing the legs, using momentum to bring the leg up and down. Keep the movement controlled.
- Focus your mind on feeling your obliques do the work.
- Hold a total contraction at the top of the movement for a count of two.
- Don't rest your leg at the bottom of the movement.

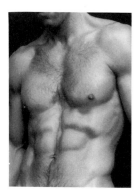

Exercise: Side Leg Raises: Both Legs

DIFFICULTY: 3
LOWER BACK: LOW RISK
AREA: OBLIQUES

STARTING POSITION: Lie on your side, resting on your left hip, both legs extended straight, and rest on your left tricep for support.

MOVEMENT: Using your oblique muscles, raise both legs off the floor as high as you can lift them. Then lower them back, lightly touching the floor. Repeat the movement until you complete your set. Then switch sides.

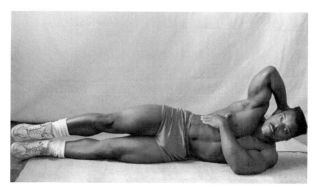

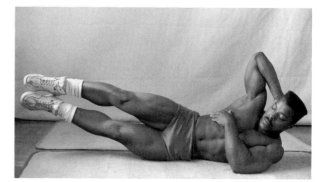

TRAINER'S TIPS:
- Concentrate on just using your ABs. Don't recruit other muscles to help you out.
- Hold a total contraction at the top of the movement for a count of two.
- Control the legs on the way down.
- Don't rest your legs on the floor at the bottom of the movement. Keep constant tension on the ABs.

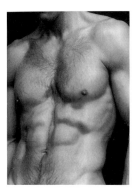

Exercise: Side Jackknife: Modified

DIFFICULTY: 1
LOWER BACK: LOW RISK
AREA: OBLIQUES

STARTING POSITION: Lie on your left hip, legs together and knees bent. Your left elbow stays close to your body for support, and your right hand goes behind your ear.

MOVEMENT: Use your oblique muscles to raise your top leg while simultaneously raising your torso to meet it. Lower in a controlled motion and repeat, until you complete your set. Then switch sides and follow the same procedure.

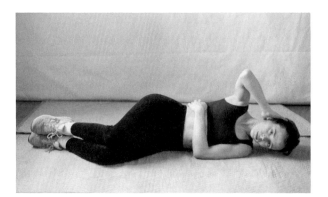

TRAINER'S TIPS:
- Focus your mind on feeling the obliques do the work.
- Make sure you get your upper body off the floor. Don't move just your head.
- Hold a total contraction at the top of the movement for a count of two.
- Don't rest your leg and your torso at the bottom of the movement.

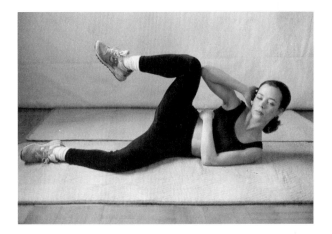

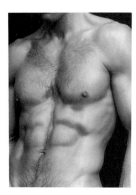

Exercise: Side Jackknife

DIFFICULTY: 2
LOWER BACK: LOW RISK
AREA: OBLIQUES (SIDES)

STARTING POSITION: Lie on your left hip, your legs together, bottom leg bent underneath for support; your right hand is behind your ear, and your left hand is placed on your right side.

MOVEMENT: Use your oblique muscle to simultaneously raise your top leg and your torso, bringing them together. Repeat the movement until you have completed your set. Then reverse procedure for opposite side.

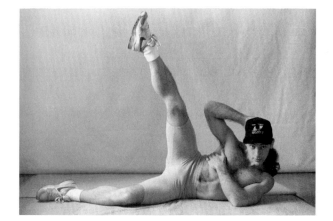

TRAINER'S TIPS:
- Bring your leg slightly forward to increase your range of motion.
- Focus your mind on feeling the obliques do the work.
- Make sure your upper body moves off the floor. Don't move just your head.
- Hold a total contraction at the top of each movement for a count of two.
- Don't rest your leg and torso at the bottom of the movement.

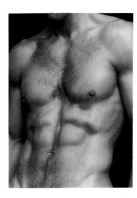

Exercise: Side Jackknife: Double Leg

DIFFICULTY: 3
LOWER BACK: MODERATE RISK
AREA: OBLIQUES

STARTING POSITION: Lie on your left hip, legs together and fully extended. Place your left elbow against your body for support and your right hand behind your ear.

MOVEMENT: Use your oblique muscles to raise both legs and simultaneously bring your torso up. Lower in a controlled motion and repeat the movement until you have completed your set. Then execute the movement on the other side.

Variation: This movement can also be done on an incline board, holding on to the board with your free hand for support.

TRAINER'S TIPS:
- Bring your legs slightly forward to increase your range of motion.
- Focus your mind on feeling the obliques do the work.
- Make sure your upper body moves off the floor. Don't move just your head.
- Hold a total contraction at the top of each movement for a count of two.

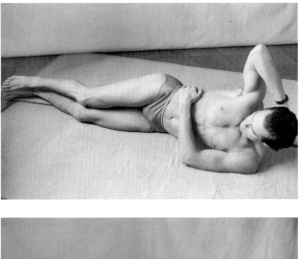

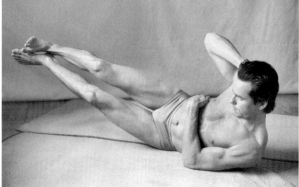

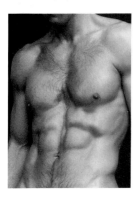

Exercise: Side Crunches

DIFFICULTY: 1
LOWER BACK: LOW RISK
AREA: OBLIQUES

STARTING POSITION: Lying on your left hip, bend your knees so they are perpendicular to your body. Put your right hand behind your head and place your left hand on your side.

MOVEMENT: In a crunchlike motion, use your obliques to lift your torso off the floor and up over your hip, bringing your rib cage toward your hip. Lower your body down so it lightly touches the floor and repeat. Reverse procedure for the opposite side.

TRAINER'S TIPS:
- Make sure you move your torso off the floor. Don't move just your head and elbow.
- Hold a total contraction at the top of the movement for a count of two.
- Focus your mind on feeling your obliques do the work.
- Make sure you get your bottom shoulder off the floor.

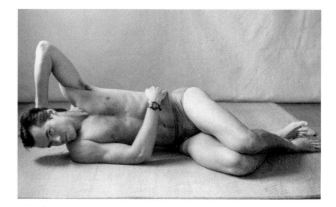

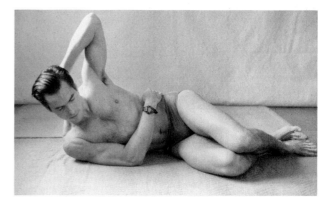

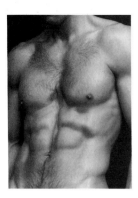

Exercise: Side Sit-ups: Roman Chair

DIFFICULTY: 3
LOWER BACK: MODERATE RISK
AREA: OBLIQUES

STARTING POSITION: Sitting on a Roman chair, rest on your left hip, hands in position of choice.

MOVEMENT: Lower your torso as close to the floor as you can, keeping your body turned to the side. Then, using your oblique muscles, raise your torso back to a sitting position (without taking tension off the ABs). Without resting, lower yourself back to the parallel position. Repeat this movement until you complete your set. Then execute the movement on the opposite side.

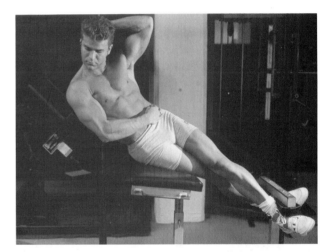

TRAINER'S TIPS:
- At the top of the movement, hold a total contraction for a count of two.
- To increase the intensity of the movement, bring your hands behind your head.
- Control the motion on the way down. Don't just drop.
- Don't rest at the top of the movement.
- Focus your mind on feeling your ABs and obliques do the work.
- Start out with Side Torso Raises or Side Jackknives before doing this movement.

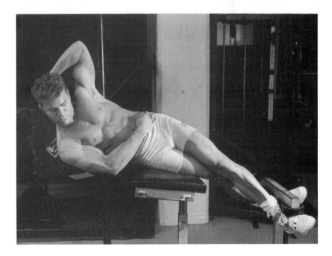

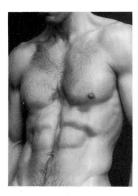

Exercise: Side Bends Without Weight

DIFFICULTY: 1
LOWER BACK: LOW RISK
AREA: OBLIQUES

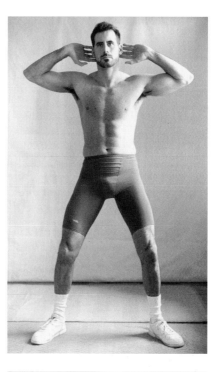

STARTING POSITION: Assume a quarter-squat position with a wide stance, feet pointed out with your hands behind your ears.

MOVEMENT: From this position, bend to the side, bringing your right elbow toward your right knee. Return to the starting position and repeat the movement until you have completed your set. Then switch sides.

TRAINER'S TIPS:
- Keep tension on the oblique throughout the movement.
- You can do this movement alternating sides or doing a set on one side, then switching sides.
- This is also a good movement to do between a series of more intense exercises.
- Focus your mind on feeling your obliques do the work.
- Hold a total contraction at the bottom of each bend for a count of two.

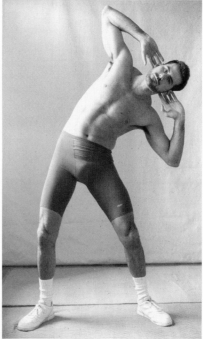

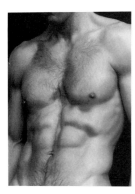

Exercise: Side Bends with Weights

DIFFICULTY: 1
LOWER BACK: MODERATE RISK
AREA: OBLIQUES

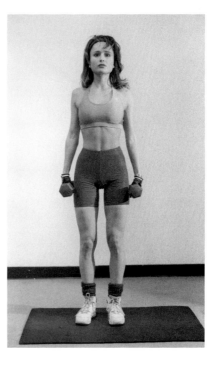

STARTING POSITION: Stand upright, feet shoulder-width apart, knees unlocked, hands at your sides holding dumbbells.

MOVEMENT: Bend to the side and lower the right dumbbell down your leg (resisting your oblique muscle) until you feel a good stretch. Then, using your oblique muscle, raise the weight back to the starting position. Then repeat the movement until you have completed your set. Then switch sides.

TRAINER'S TIPS:
- Keep the obliques flexed throughout the movement.
- Concentrate on feeling your obliques raise and lower the weight.
- Using heavy weights will build muscle mass. So you will probably want to use light weights and do this exercise only periodically.
- Don't rest at the top of the movement.

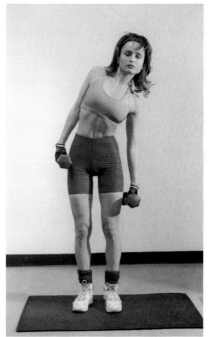

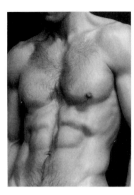

Exercise: Seated Twists

DIFFICULTY: 1
LOWER BACK: LOW RISK
AREA: OBLIQUES

STARTING POSITION: Sit on a bench, feet flat on the floor, spread wide apart for support, holding a light bar or broom handle across your shoulders.

MOVEMENT: Keeping your hips stationary, use your oblique muscles to twist your torso to the left as far as it can go, and then twist back to the right through a full range of motion.

TRAINER'S TIPS:
- Keep a slow, controlled motion at the beginning of your set. Then, as you get looser, you can pick up the pace.
- Don't jerk from side to side.
- Remain in constant motion during this exercise.
- If you have lower-back problems, keep the movement slow and controlled throughout.

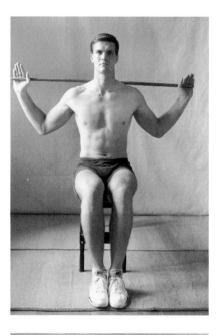

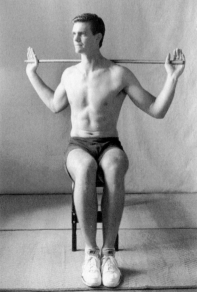

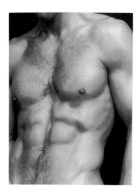

Exercise: Standing Twists

DIFFICULTY: 1
LOWER BACK: LOW RISK
AREA: OBLIQUE

STARTING POSITION: Stand upright, feet a little wider than shoulder width, knees unlocked, holding a broom handle or light bar across the top of your shoulders.

MOVEMENT: Keeping your hips stationary, use your oblique muscles to twist your torso to the left as far as it can go, and then twist back to the right through a full range of motion.

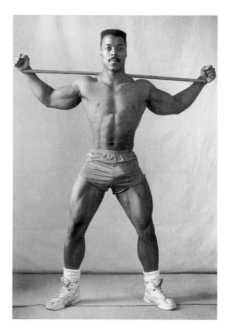

TRAINER'S TIPS:
- Keep a slow, controlled motion at the beginning of your set. Then, as you get looser, you can pick up the pace.
- Don't turn your hips. Keep them stable. Your range of movement will be determined by how far you can twist without letting your hips start to turn.
- If you have lower-back problems, you should keep the motion slow and controlled.
- Keep in constant motion during this movement.

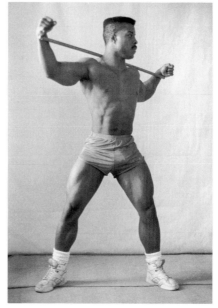

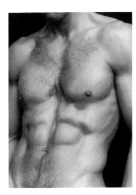

Exercise: Standing Twists: Bent Over

DIFFICULTY: 1
LOWER BACK: LOW RISK
AREA: OBLIQUES

STARTING POSITION: Stand upright, feet a little wider than shoulder width, knees unlocked, holding a light bar or broom handle across your shoulders. Then bend forward at the waist to a comfortable position. A good guideline is to have your upper body at about a 45-degree angle.

MOVEMENT: Keeping your hips stationary, use the oblique muscles to twist to the right, bringing the broom handle vertical, and then back to the left through a full range of motion. Continue to repeat the movement until you have completed your set.

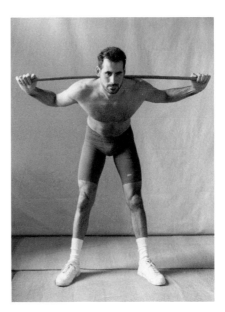

> **TRAINER'S TIPS:**
> • Start out with a slow, controlled motion, then you can speed it up as your body becomes looser and your muscles warm up.
> • Don't turn your hips. Keep them stable. Your range of movement will be determined by how far you can twist without letting your hips turn.
> • Keep the motion constant during this exercise.

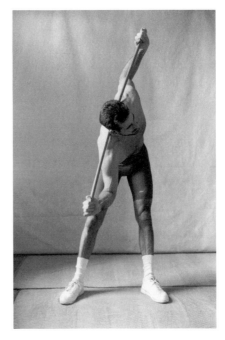

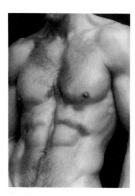

Exercise: Leg Overs: Bent-Knee, Single Leg

DIFFICULTY: 1
LOWER BACK: LOW RISK
AREA: OBLIQUES

STARTING POSITION: Lie flat on your back, hands spread out perpendicular to your body, left leg fully extended, and your right knee bent at a 90-degree angle to the body, with your lower leg extended out.

MOVEMENT: Use your oblique muscles to cross your right knee over your body, lightly touching the floor on the opposite side. Then cross it back over to the starting position. Repeat this movement until you complete your set. Then switch legs.

TRAINER'S TIPS:
- As you cross your leg over, allow your hip to roll with the motion.
- Concentrate on feeling your obliques do the work.
- Make sure you keep the lower half of your leg extended out during the movement.
- Keep both shoulder blades on the floor throughout the movement.
- Think of having the leg, hip, and oblique muscle fused together, so they move as a single unit.

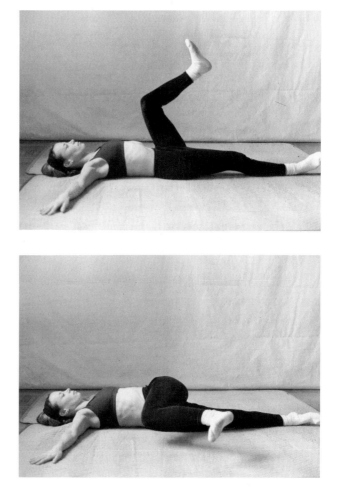

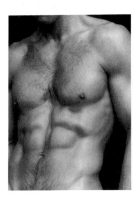

Exercise: Leg Overs: Single Leg

DIFFICULTY: 1
LOWER BACK: LOW RISK
AREA: OBLIQUES

STARTING POSITION: Lie flat on your back, hands spread out perpendicular to your body, left leg fully extended, right leg straight up.

MOVEMENT: Use your oblique muscles to cross your right leg toward your left hand. Lightly touch the floor with your foot, then cross the leg back to the straight-up starting position. Repeat this movement until you complete your set. Then switch legs.

TRAINER'S TIPS:
- As you cross the leg over, allow your hip to roll with the motion.
- Concentrate on feeling your ABs do the work.
- If you can't move your leg to the straight-up position or over close to your hand, just move it to a position that is comfortable. Your flexibility will improve.
- Think of having the leg, hip, and oblique muscle fused together, so they move as a single unit.
- Keep both shoulder blades on the floor throughout the movement.

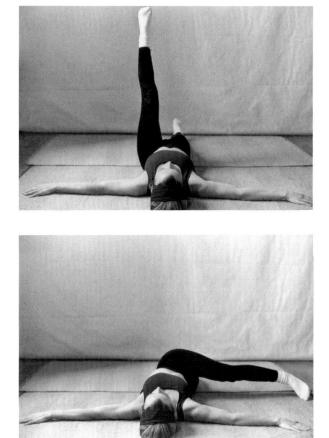

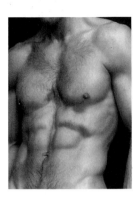

Exercise: Leg Overs: Bent-Knee, Double Leg

DIFFICULTY: 2
LOWER BACK: LOW RISK
AREA: OBLIQUES

STARTING POSITION: Lie flat on your back, hands spread out perpendicular to your body, both knees up, lower legs extended out.

MOVEMENT: Use your oblique muscles to lower both legs to your left side, so that your lower leg lightly touches the floor, then raise them back to the starting position. Then repeat the movement to the opposite side.

TRAINER'S TIPS:
- As you lower your legs to the side, let your hips roll in the direction with the motion.
- Concentrate on feeling your AB muscles do the work.
- Keep your lower legs extended throughout the movement.
- Keep both shoulder blades on the floor throughout the movement.

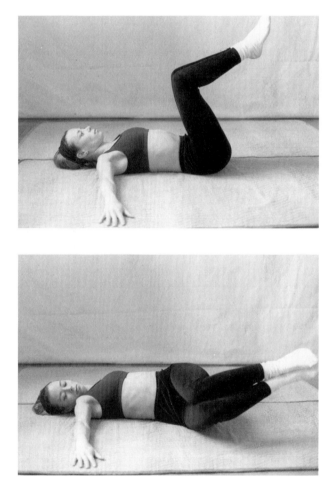

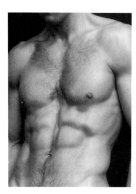

Exercise: Leg Overs: Double Leg

DIFFICULTY: 3
LOWER BACK: MODERATE RISK
AREA: OBLIQUES

STARTING POSITION: Lie flat on your back, hands spread out perpendicular to your body, with both legs extended straight up.

MOVEMENT: Use your oblique muscles to resist as you lower both legs to your left side until your feet lightly touch the floor, then raise them back to the starting position. Repeat the movement to the opposite side.

TRAINER'S TIPS:
- As you lower both legs to the side, let your hips roll in that direction with the motion.
- Try to lower your legs at a 90-degree angle from your upper body.
- If you can't move your legs to the straight-up position or lower them at a 90-degree angle, take them to a level angle that is comfortable. Your flexibility will improve.
- Keep your shoulders and back flat on the floor throughout the entire movement.
- Concentrate on feeling your AB muscles do the work.
- This movement is the most difficult of the Leg-Over series, so work up to it gradually building strength with the other movements first.

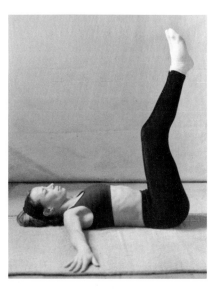

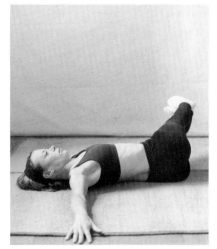

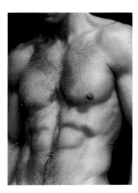

Exercise: Hip-ups

DIFFICULTY: 3
LOWER BACK: MODERATE RISK
AREA: OBLIQUES

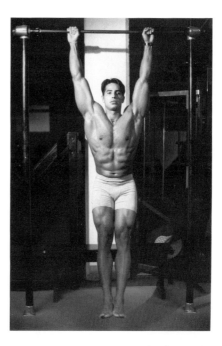

STARTING POSITION: Hang from a bar or vertical chair, legs fully extended.

MOVEMENT: Rotate your hip clockwise, raise your knees perpendicular to your body, then raise your hips toward your rib cage. Lower your knees back to starting position. Repeat the movement to the opposite side. Continue the movement until you complete your set.

TRAINER'S TIPS:
- Don't let your legs rest at the bottom of the movement.
- Hold a total contraction at the top of the movement.
- Don't swing to gain momentum.
- Control the motion on the way down. Don't just let your hip drop.
- Focus your mind on feeling your obliques lift your hip.
- If you can't get your hip up very high, just go as high as you can. Your range of motion will improve with work.

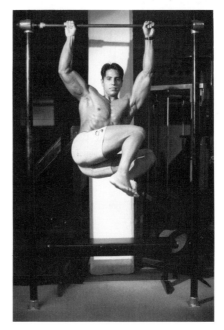

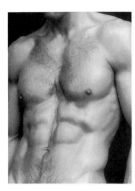

Exercise: Elbow to Hip

DIFFICULTY: 1
LOWER BACK: LOW RISK
AREA: OBLIQUES

STARTING POSITION: Lie flat on your back, knees bent, feet flat on the floor, and left hand behind your ear.

MOVEMENT: Use your oblique muscles to bend your elbow to your hip. Then straighten your torso back to the starting position. Repeat the movement until you complete your set. Follow the same procedure for the opposite side.

TRAINER'S TIPS:
- Focus your mind on feeling the oblique muscles bend the body.
- Hold a total contraction for a count of two as the elbow meets the hip.
- Keep your elbow close to the floor as you make a semicircle toward your hip.

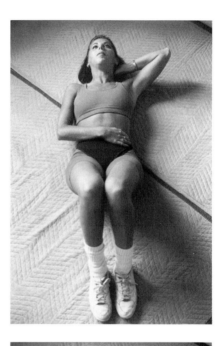

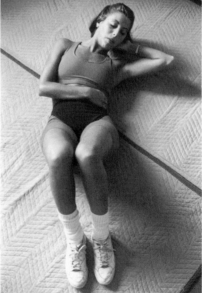

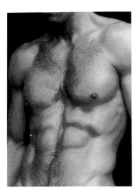

Exercise: Raised Side Bends with a Cross

DIFFICULTY: 3
LOWER BACK: MODERATE RISK
AREA: OBLIQUES

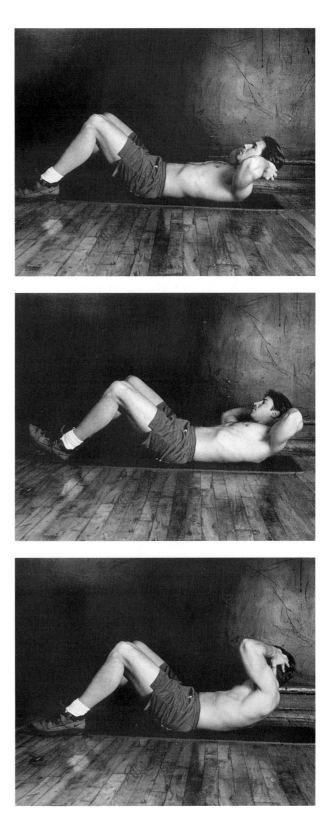

STARTING POSITION: Lie on your back, knees up, feet flat on the floor, head and neck relaxed.

MOVEMENT: Raise your shoulder blades off the floor, then bend at the waist, moving to your right laterally just above the floor, bringing the side of your right rib cage toward your right hip. When you've moved that direction as far as you can, cross your left shoulder toward your right knee. Repeat this movement in the opposite direction.

TRAINER'S TIPS:
- The movement from side to side is the same as a standing side bend, except you are lying down.
- Move as far to the left and right as you can.
- Keep your shoulder blades off the floor for the entire exercise.
- The crossing movement is a small diagonal movement.
- Focus your mind on your obliques.

CHAPTER TWELVE

Area Three: The Upper ABs

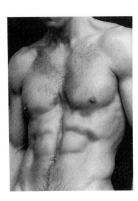

Exercise: Crunches: Knees Bent

DIFFICULTY: 1
LOWER BACK: LOW RISK
AREA: UPPER ABS

STARTING POSITION: Lie on your back, knees bent so your feet rest flat on the floor, and your hands in position of choice.

MOVEMENT: Use your upper ABs to raise your shoulder blades off the floor in a forward-curling motion. Then lower your shoulders to the starting position, lightly touching your shoulder blades to the floor. Repeat.

Variation: You can also do the crunch movement on an incline board.

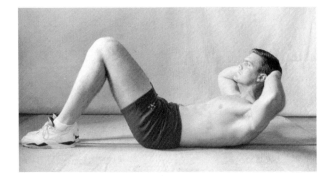

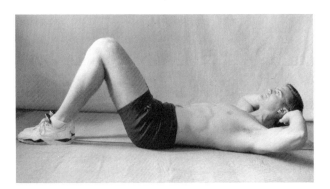

TRAINER'S TIPS:
- Keep constant tension on your ABs throughout the movement.
- Focus your mind on feeling your upper ABs do the work.
- Don't rest at the bottom of the movement.
- Hold a total contraction at the top of the movement for a count of two.
- Make sure you move your shoulders off the floor. Don't move just your neck and head.
- Keep the small of your back pressed against the floor.

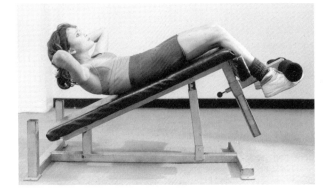

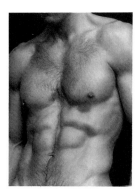

Exercise: Crunches: Knees Up

DIFFICULTY: 1
LOWER BACK: LOW RISK
AREA: UPPER ABS

STARTING POSITION: Lie on your back and raise your legs so your thighs are perpendicular to your body, placing your calves and feet parallel to the floor and hands in position of choice.

MOVEMENT: Use the muscles of your upper ABs to raise your shoulders and back off the floor in a forward-curling motion. Then lower your torso to the starting position, lightly touching your shoulder blades to the floor. Repeat.

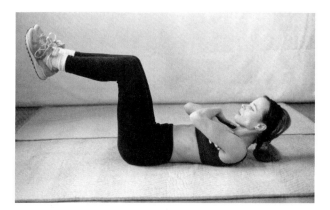

TRAINER'S TIPS:
- Get your shoulders off the floor with each repetition. Don't move just your neck up and down.
- Keep the movement controlled.
- Hold a total contraction at the top of each movement for a count of two.
- Don't rest your shoulders on the floor at the bottom of the movement.
- Focus your mind on feeling your upper ABs do the work.
- Keep the small of your back pressed against the floor.

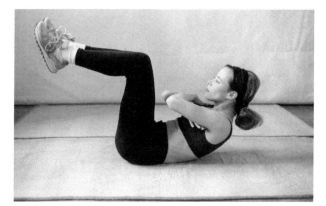

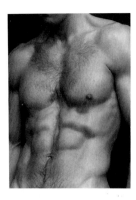

Exercise: Crunches: Legs Straight Up

DIFFICULTY: 2
LOWER BACK: LOW RISK
AREA: UPPER ABS

STARTING POSITION: Lie on your back, legs straight up perpendicular to your body (knees unlocked), head up, and hands in position of choice.

MOVEMENT: Use the muscles of your upper ABs to raise your shoulders and back off the floor in a forward-curling motion. Then lower your torso to the starting position, lightly touching your shoulder blades to the floor. Repeat.

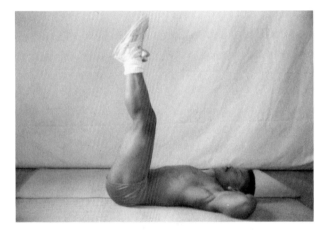

TRAINER'S TIPS:
- Keep constant tension on the ABs throughout the movement.
- Focus your mind on feeling your upper ABs do the work.
- Don't rest at the bottom of the movement.
- Hold a total contraction at the top of the movement for a count of two.
- Make sure you move your shoulders off the floor. Don't move just your neck and head.
- Keep the movement controlled. Don't do it too fast, turning it into a rocking motion.
- Don't raise your hips off the floor to help bring your legs perpendicular. This will activate your lower ABs and inhibit the movement in your upper ABs.
- Keep small of back pressed against the floor.

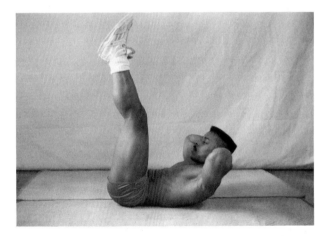

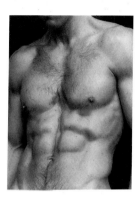

Exercise: Toe Touches

DIFFICULTY: 2
LOWER BACK: MODERATE RISK
AREA: UPPER ABS

STARTING POSITION: Lie flat on your back, legs straight up, perpendicular to your body (knees unlocked), and arms extended parallel to your body.

MOVEMENT: Use your upper ABs to raise your hands to your toes. Then lower your shoulders, letting your shoulder blades lightly touch the floor. Repeat the movement until you complete your set.

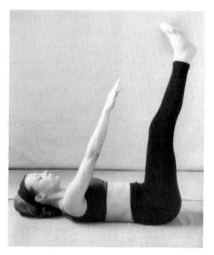

TRAINER'S TIPS:
- Focus your mind on feeling the upper ABs do the work.
- Don't rest at the bottom of the movement. When you feel your shoulders touch, start the next repetition.
- If you can't touch your toes, just reach as far as you can. Your range of movement will improve with time and work.
- Hold a total contraction at the top of the movement for a count of two.
- If you have problems getting your legs perpendicular, have a partner hold them or sit against the wall.
- Variation: Bring your legs as close to perpendicular as possible, reaching your hands to the ceiling, instead of angling toward your toes.
- Keep small of back pressed against the floor.

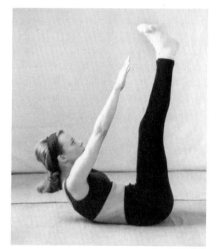

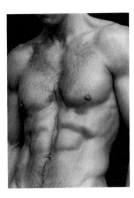

Exercise: Crunches: Legs Straight Out

DIFFICULTY: 2
LOWER BACK: MODERATE RISK
AREA: UPPER ABS

STARTING POSITION: Lie on your back, feet extended straight out on the floor (knees unlocked) and hands in position of choice.

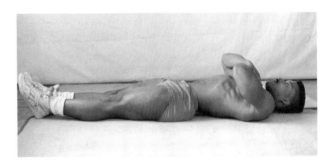

MOVEMENT: Use the muscles of your upper ABs to raise your shoulders and back off the floor in a forward-curling motion. Then lower your shoulders to the starting position, lightly touching your shoulder blades to the floor. Repeat.

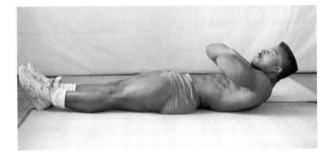

TRAINER'S TIPS:
- Make sure you keep your knees unlocked so your thigh muscles aren't contracting.
- Turn your knees slightly out.
- Keep constant tension on the ABs throughout the movement.
- Don't rest at the bottom of the movement.
- Hold a total contraction at the top of the movement for a count of two.
- Focus your mind on feeling your upper ABs do the work.
- Make sure you move your shoulders off the floor. Don't move just the neck and head.
- Try to keep your lower back pressed against the floor.

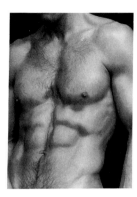

Exercise: Crunches: Frog Legs

DIFFICULTY: 1
LOWER BACK: LOW RISK
AREA: UPPER ABS

STARTING POSITION: Lying on your back, bring the soles of your feet together, keeping your feet on the ground and your knees flattened out. Place hands in position of choice.

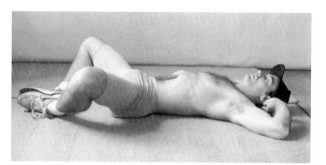

MOVEMENT: Using the muscles of your upper ABs, raise your shoulders and upper back off the floor. Then lower your shoulders to starting position, lightly touching the floor. Repeat.

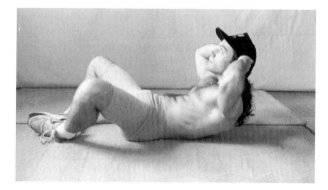

TRAINER'S TIPS:
• Keep constant tension on your ABs.
• Focus your mind on your upper ABs, feeling them do the work.
• Don't rest at the bottom of the movement.
• Hold a total contraction at the top of the movement for a count of two.
• Make sure you move your shoulder off the floor. Don't move just your neck and head.
• Keep your lower back pressed against the floor.
• As in other crunch variations, this leg position adds variety and hits the muscle from a different angle, shocking the muscle and giving it better overall development.

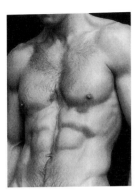

Exercise: Crunches: Raised Hip

DIFFICULTY: 2
LOWER BACK: MODERATE RISK
AREA: UPPER ABS

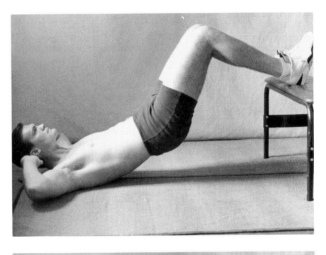

STARTING POSITION: Lie on your back, knees bent, feet extended out at a 90-degree angle and pressed up against a wall or bench. Keep your head up and place your hands in position of choice. Push your hips up toward the ceiling (about six inches off the floor), so your buttocks are contracted. Hold this position throughout the exercise.

MOVEMENT: Use your upper ABs to raise your shoulders off the floor. Lower and repeat. You will probably get only one to three inches of movement, so don't be discouraged.

TRAINER'S TIPS:
- Keep constant tension on your ABs throughout the movement.
- Focus your mind on your upper ABs, feeling them do the work.
- Don't rest at the bottom of the movement.
- Hold a total contraction at the top of the movement for a count of two.
- Make sure you move your shoulders off the floor. Don't move just your neck and head.
- Keep the movement controlled.

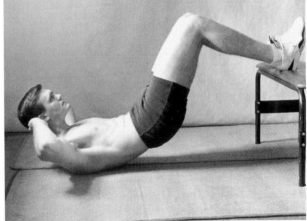

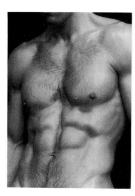

Exercise: Crunches: Split Leg

DIFFICULTY: 1
LOWER BACK: MODERATE RISK
AREA: UPPER ABS AND OBLIQUES

START: Lie flat on your back, left leg straight up perpendicular to your body (knee unlocked), right leg extended on the floor (knee unlocked), and hands in position of choice.

MOVEMENT: Use your AB muscles to raise your chest toward your left knee in a curling motion. Then lower yourself until your shoulder blades lightly touch the floor. Repeat.

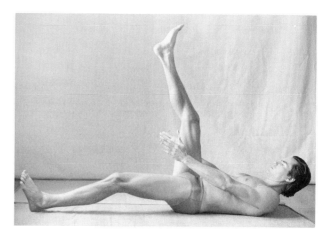

TRAINER'S TIPS:
- Hold a total contraction at the top of the movement for a count of two.
- Get your shoulder blades off the floor with each repetition. Don't move just your head and neck.
- Don't rest at the bottom of the movement. When you feet your shoulder blades touch, start the next repetition.
- Focus your mind on feeling your ABs do the work.
- Keep small of back pressed against floor and maintain stable position—do not rock.

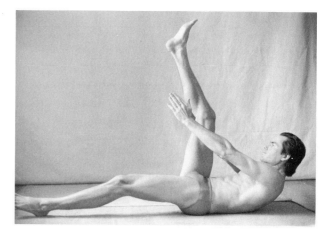

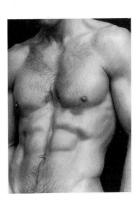

Exercise: Crunches: Knees Bent, Spread

DIFFICULTY: 1
LOWER BACK: LOW RISK
AREA: UPPER ABS

STARTING POSITION: Lie on your back, knees bent so your feet rest flat on the floor and your hands in position of choice. Then spread your legs wide.

MOVEMENT: Use your upper ABs to raise your shoulder blades off the floor in a forward-curling motion. Then lower your shoulders to the starting position, lightly touching your shoulder blades to the floor. Repeat.

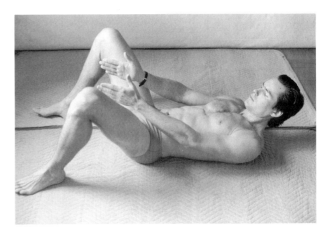

TRAINER'S TIPS:
- Keep constant tension on your ABs throughout the movement.
- Focus your mind on feeling your upper ABs do the work.
- Don't rest at the bottom of the movement.
- Hold a total contraction at the top of the movement for a count of two.
- Make sure you move your shoulders off the floor. Don't move just your neck and head.
- Keep the small of your back pressed against the floor.

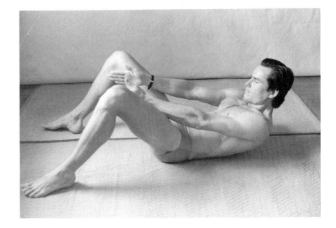

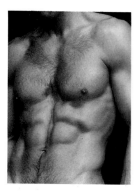

Exercise: Crunches: Knees Up, Spread

DIFFICULTY: 1
LOWER BACK: LOW RISK
AREA: UPPER ABS

STARTING POSITION: Lie on your back, raise your legs so your thighs are perpendicular to your body, placing your calves and feet parallel to the floor and hands in position of choice. Then spread your legs wide.

MOVEMENT: Use the muscles of your upper ABs to raise your shoulders and back off the floor in a forward-curling motion. Then lower your torso to the starting position, lightly touching your shoulder blades to the floor. Repeat.

TRAINER'S TIPS:
- Get your shoulders off the floor with each repetition. Don't move just your neck up and down.
- Keep the movement controlled.
- Hold a total contraction at the top of each movement for a count of two.
- Don't rest your shoulders on the floor at the bottom of the movement.
- Focus your mind on feeling your upper ABs do the work.

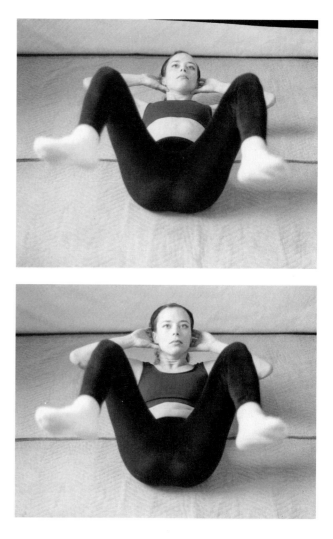

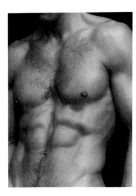

Exercise: Crunches: Legs Straight Out, Spread

DIFFICULTY: 2
LOWER BACK: MODERATE RISK
AREA: UPPER ABS

STARTING POSITION: Lie on your back, feet extended straight out on the floor (knees unlocked) and hands in position of choice. Then spread your legs wide.

MOVEMENT: Use the muscles of your upper ABs to raise your shoulders and back off the floor in a forward-curling motion. Then lower your shoulders to the starting position, lightly touching your shoulder blades to the floor.

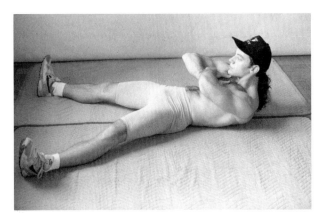

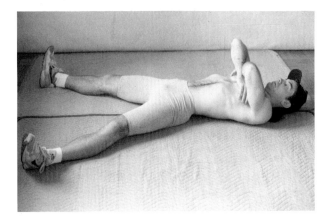

TRAINER'S TIPS:
- Make sure you keep your knees unlocked so your thigh muscles aren't contracting.
- Turn your knees slightly out.
- Keep constant tension on the ABs throughout the movement.
- Don't rest at the bottom of the movement.
- Hold a total contraction at the top of the movement for a count of two.
- Focus your mind on feeling your upper ABs do the work.
- Make sure you move your shoulders off the floor. Don't move just the neck and head.

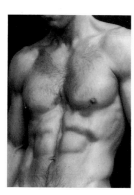

Exercise: Bench Crunches

DIFFICULTY: 2
LOWER BACK: MODERATE RISK
AREA: UPPER ABS

STARTING POSITION: Lie on your back on a bench, bending your knees, placing both feet flat on the bench. Then position your shoulder blades so they drop over the edge of the bench, and support your head with the hand position of choice.

MOVEMENT: Use your upper ABs to raise and curl your torso up and over the bench toward your rib cage. Then lower your shoulders below the bench and repeat.

TRAINER'S TIPS:
- Keep constant tension on your ABs throughout the full range of motion (both raising and lowering).
- Make sure you lower your shoulders below the bench on each repetition.
- Raise the torso as high as you would on a normal crunch.
- Don't rest at the bottom of the movement.
- Focus your mind on your upper ABs.

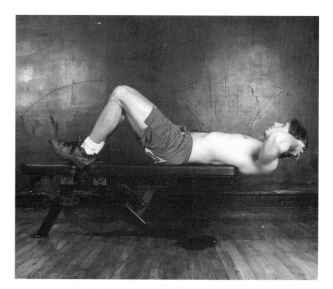

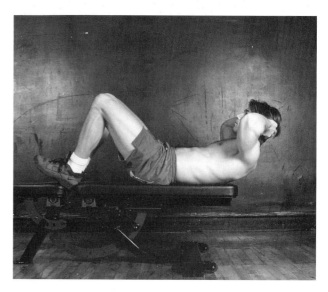

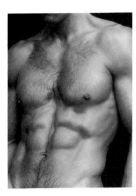

Exercise: Cable Crunches

DIFFICULTY: 3
LOWER BACK: LOW RISK
AREA: UPPER ABS

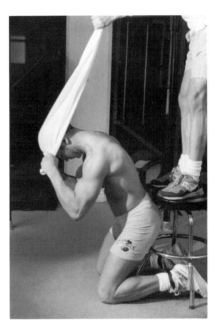

STARTING POSITION: Grab the cable attachment of a pulldown or use a towel with a partner giving you manual resistance (see photo). Kneel facing the cable machine, hips up, holding the attachment to your forehead with both hands.

MOVEMENT: Use your upper ABs to bend forward. Bring your head down and out over your knees, driving your elbows to your knees while keeping the cable tight and held stationary at your forehead. Come up to approximately a 45-degree angle. Repeat.

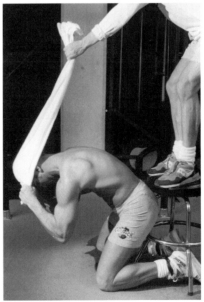

TRAINER'S TIPS:
- Raise and lower the weights in a controlled motion. Don't pop back up.
- Don't come all the way up on each repetition—maintain approximately the 45-degree angle.
- Hold a total contraction at the bottom of the movement.
- Imagine that you are bending over a bar that is about six inches from your body at stomach level.
- Hold a total contraction at the bottom of the movement for a count of two.

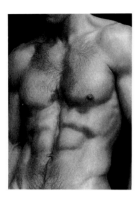

Exercise: Crunches: Legs Straight Up, Spread

DIFFICULTY: 2
LOWER BACK: LOW RISK
AREA: UPPER ABS

STARTING POSITION: Lie on your back, legs straight up perpendicular to your body (knees unlocked), head up, and hands in position of choice. Then spread your legs wide.

MOVEMENT: Use the muscles of your upper ABs to raise your shoulders and back off the floor in a forward-curling motion. Then lower your torso to the starting position, lightly touching your shoulder blades to the floor. Repeat.

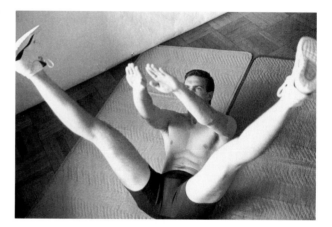

TRAINER'S TIPS:
- Keep constant tension on the ABs throughout the movement.
- Focus your mind on feeling your upper ABs do the work.
- Don't rest at the bottom of the movement.
- Hold a total contraction at the top of the movement for a count of two.
- Make sure you move your shoulders off the floor. Don't move just your neck and head.
- Keep the movement controlled. Don't do it too fast, turning it into a rocking motion.
- Don't raise your hips off the floor to help bring your legs perpendicular. This will activate your lower ABs and inhibit the movement in your upper ABs.
- Keep your lower back pressed against the floor.

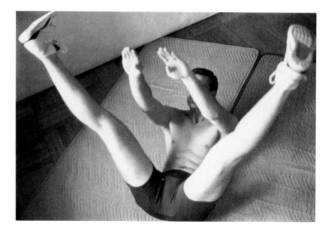

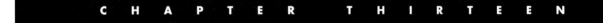

CHAPTER THIRTEEN

Area Four:
Combination
Exercises

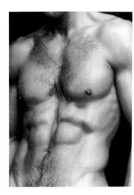

Exercise: Crossovers

DIFFICULTY: 2
LOWER BACK: LOW RISK
AREA: UPPER AND LOWER ABS
AND OBLIQUES

STARTING POSITION: Lie on your back, knees up and both feet on the floor. Then cross your left leg over the right leg. Your ankle should rest just below the knee, making a triangle between your legs. Keep your left leg away from your torso. Your right hand goes behind your ear, elbow straight out. Both your head and elbow are resting on the floor. Place your left hand on your right side.

MOVEMENT: Use your ABs to raise and twist your right shoulder toward your opposite knee. Then lower your torso back to the floor. Repeat. Then reverse the procedure for the other side.

TRAINER'S TIPS:
- Make sure your entire torso twists toward your knee. Don't move just the elbow. And don't move your knee.
- Focus your mind on feeling your ABs do the work.
- Don't rest at the bottom of the movement—keep constant tension on the ABs.
- Keep small of back pressed against floor and maintain stable position. Do not rock.

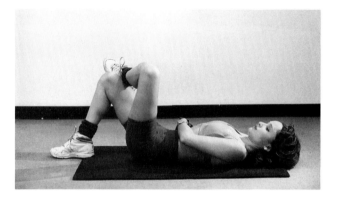

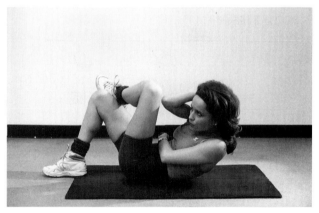

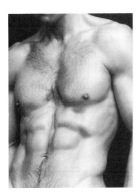

Exercise: Bicycles

DIFFICULTY: 2
LOWER BACK: MODERATE RISK
AREA: UPPER AND LOWER ABS
AND OBLIQUES

STARTING POSITION: Lie on your back, thighs perpendicular to your torso, feet parallel to the floor, and your hands behind your ears.

MOVEMENT: Use your ABs to simultaneously bring your right shoulder and your left knee together (so your elbow meets your knee). Then extend your left leg at an approximately 45-degree angle from the floor, as you cross your left shoulder to your right knee (elbow meeting knee). Repeat in a fluid motion to the other side. Keep the motion continuous, as if you were pedaling a bicycle.

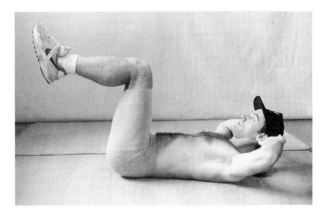

TRAINER'S TIPS:
- Keep the motion controlled. Don't go too fast.
- Make sure your entire torso twists. Don't move just the elbow to the knee.
- Make sure your shoulder blades come off the floor each time.
- Don't let your legs touch the floor.
- Focus your mind on feeling your ABs do the work.
- Keep the small of your back pressed against the floor and maintain a stable position. Do not rock.

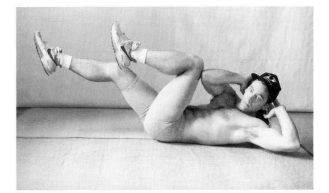

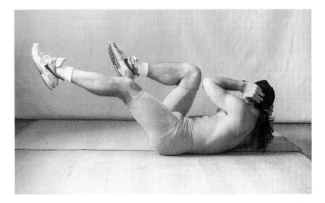

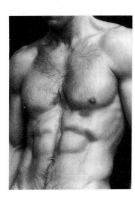

Exercise: Double Crunch

DIFFICULTY: 2
LOWER BACK: MODERATE RISK
AREA: UPPER AND LOWER ABS

STARTING POSITION: Lie flat on your back, the lower part of your right leg resting on your left knee. Raise your left leg slightly off the floor.

MOVEMENT: Use your ABs to simultaneously raise your hips and shoulder blades off the floor and toward each other.

TRAINER'S TIPS:
- Your foot should not touch the ground during the exercise.
- The small of your back should remain pressed against the floor during the entire exercise.
- The leg that is resting on top of the knee should be pointed straight back and not flared out.
- Focus your mind on feeling your ABs do the work.
- Hold a total contraction for a count of two at the top of the movement.

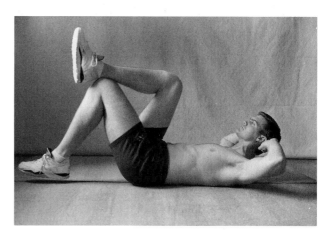

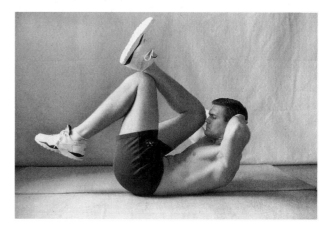

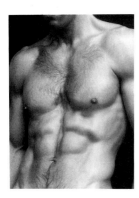

Exercise: Corkscrews

DIFFICULTY: 3
LOWER BACK: MODERATE RISK
AREA: LOWER ABS AND OBLIQUES

STARTING POSITION: Lie flat on your back, legs straight up and perpendicular to your body, and hands at your sides, palms flat.

MOVEMENT: Use your ABs to elevate your hips off the ground, pushing your legs straight up and twisting your hips in a corkscrew motion. First twist them clockwise, lowering your hips until they lightly touch the floor. Then twist counterclockwise and lower. Keep alternating until you have completed your set. Each twist equals a repetition.

TRAINER'S TIPS:
- Keep constant tension on your ABs.
- Focus your mind on feeling your ABs do the work.
- Don't rest at the bottom of the movement.
- Hold a total contraction at the top of the movement for a count of two.
- Don't kick up with your legs to elevate the hips—keep the movement controlled.
- Press your hands against the floor for stability. Don't press off your fingertips.
- Return to perpendicular leg position after each repetition. Do not bring legs and feet to floor.

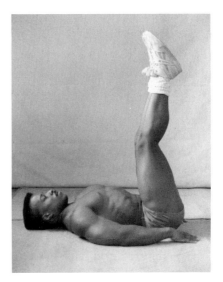

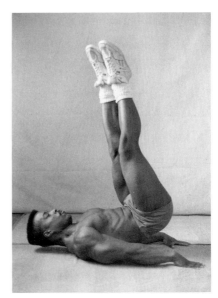

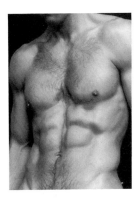

Exercise: Circles

DIFFICULTY: 2
LOWER BACK: MODERATE RISK
AREA: UPPER ABS AND OBLIQUES

STARTING POSITION: Lie flat on your back, knees bent so your feet rest flat on the floor, with your hands in position of choice.

MOVEMENT: Use your upper ABs to curl your torso toward your rib cage in a small circular motion. If your torso was a hand on a clock, starting position would be six o'clock; moving up and around to twelve o'clock (position of a normal crunch) and back down and around to six o'clock completes one repetition. Alternate directions with each repetition.

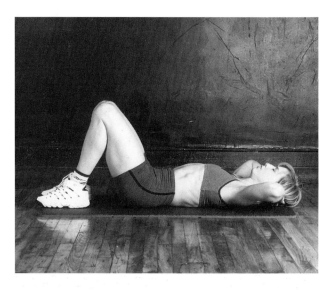

TRAINER'S TIPS:
- Keep constant tension on your ABs throughout the full range of motion (all directions).
- Raise your torso as high as you would on a normal crunch.
- Don't rest at the bottom of the movement.
- Focus your mind on your ABs.

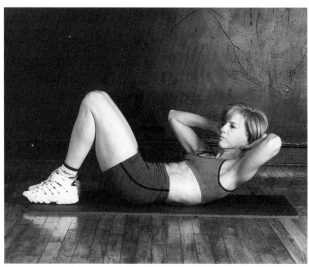

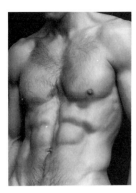

Exercise: Reverse Crunch Circles

DIFFICULTY: 3
LOWER BACK: MODERATE RISK
AREA: LOWER ABS AND OBLIQUES

STARTING POSITION: Lie flat on your back, positioning your legs so your thighs are perpendicular to your body and your lower legs are parallel to the floor.

MOVEMENT: Use your lower ABs to curl your hips toward your rib cage in a small circular motion. If your hips were a hand on a clock, starting position would be six o'clock; moving up and around to twelve o'clock (position of a normal reverse crunch) and back down and around to six o'clock completes one repetition. Alternate directions with each repetition.

TRAINER'S TIPS:
- Keep constant tension on your ABs throughout the full range of motion (all directions).
- Raise the hips as high as you would on a normal reverse crunch.
- Don't rest at the bottom of the movement.
- Focus your mind on your ABs.

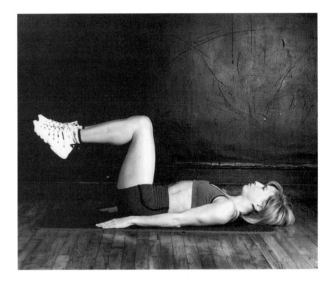

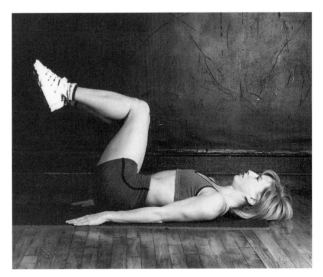

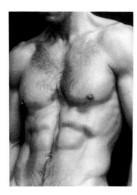

Exercise: Elbows to Knees

DIFFICULTY: 2
LOWER BACK: MODERATE RISK
AREA: LOWER AND UPPER ABS

STARTING POSITION: Lie flat on your back, knees bent, feet flat on the floor, and hands behind your ears, elbows forward.

MOVEMENT: Use your ABs to simultaneously raise your torso and your legs until your elbows touch your knees. Lower back to the starting position. Repeat.

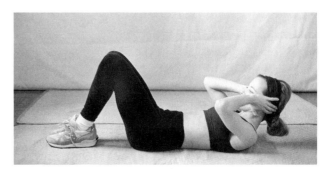

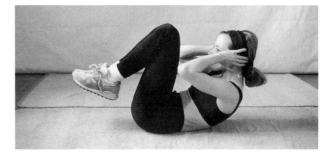

TRAINER'S TIPS:
- Concentrate on keeping constant tension on the ABs.
- Focus your mind on feeling your ABs do the work.
- Hold a total contraction for a count of two when the knees and elbows meet.
- Don't let the shoulders or feet rest on the floor at the completion of each repetition.
- Let your heels lightly touch the ground on each rep.
- Don't bring your knees forward and have your elbows meet your knees at the midpoint of the movement.
- Keep lower back firmly pressed to the floor through both ranges of motion (raising and lowering).

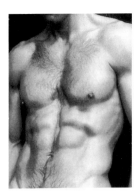

Exercise: Elbows to Knee: Single Leg, Bent

DIFFICULTY: 1
LOWER BACK: MODERATE RISK
AREA: UPPER AND LOWER ABS

STARTING POSITION: Lie flat on your back, knees bent, feet flat on the floor, and hands behind your ears.

MOVEMENT: Use your ABs to simultaneously raise your left knee and torso, bringing both elbows to the knee. Then lower your upper body and leg back to starting position. Repeat the movement to the opposite side. Continue to alternate until you complete your set.

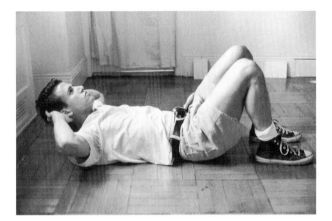

TRAINER'S TIPS:
- Keep constant tension on the ABs.
- Focus your mind on feeling your ABs do the work.
- Hold a total contraction for a count of two when the elbows meet the knee.
- Don't let the shoulders and leg rest on the floor at the bottom of each repetition.
- You can do all your repetitions on one leg, then switch, or alternate legs.
- Keep small of back pressed against the ground and maintain a stable position—do not rock.

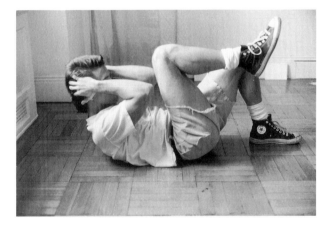

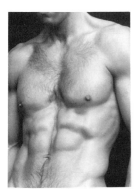

Exercise: Elbows to Knee: Single Leg, Straight

DIFFICULTY: 2
LOWER BACK: HIGH RISK
AREA: UPPER AND LOWER ABS

STARTING POSITION: Lie flat on your back, legs fully extended (knees unlocked), heels on the floor, hands in position of choice.

MOVEMENT: Use your ABs to simultaneously raise your right leg (to at least perpendicular with your torso) and bring both elbows to your knee. Then lower upper body and leg back to the starting position. Repeat the movement to the opposite side.

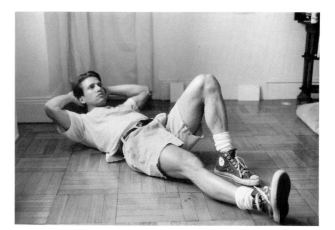

TRAINER'S TIPS:
- You can do all your repetitions on one side or alternate.
- Keep constant tension on the ABs.
- Focus your mind on feeling the ABs do the work.
- Hold a total contraction for a count of two when the elbows meet the knee.
- Don't let your shoulders and your leg rest on the floor at the bottom of each repetition.
- Keep your knee unlocked throughout the movement.
- Keep small of back pressed against floor and maintain a stable position—do not rock.

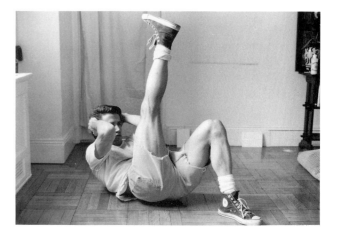

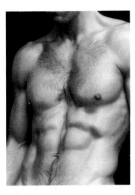

Exercise: Elbow to Knees: Bent-Knee Cross

DIFFICULTY: 2
LOWER BACK: MODERATE RISK
AREA: LOWER AND UPPER ABS
AND OBLIQUES

STARTING POSITION: Lie flat on your back, knees bent, feet flat on the floor, right hand behind your right ear, and left hand at your side.

MOVEMENT: Use your ABs to simultaneously raise your right shoulder and your left leg off the floor (knee bent), crossing them toward each other, until your knee and elbow meet in the middle of the movement. Lower them back to the starting position. Repeat.

TRAINER'S TIPS:
- Keep constant tension on the ABs.
- Focus your mind on feeling your ABs do the work.
- Hold a total contraction when the knee and elbows meet for a count of two.
- Don't let the shoulders or foot rest on the floor at the completion of each repetition.
- Keep the knee bent throughout the movement.
- Keep your lower back pressed to ground to maintain solid base. Do not rock or jerk.

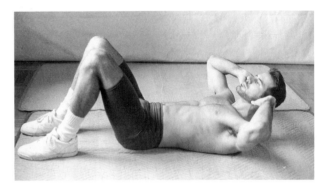

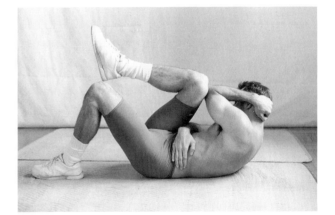

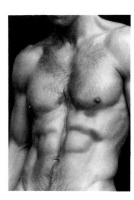

Exercise: Elbow to Knees: Straight-Leg Cross

DIFFICULTY: 2
LOWER BACK: HIGH RISK
AREA: RECTUS ABDOMINIS AND OBLIQUES

STARTING POSITION: Lie on your back, right knee bent, left leg extended straight (knees unlocked), right hand behind your ear, and your left hand at your side.

MOVEMENT: Use your ABs to simultaneously raise your left leg and bring your right shoulder off the floor, crossing them toward each other, the elbow meeting the knee in the middle of the movement. Then lower your shoulder and leg back to the starting position. Repeat.

TRAINER'S TIPS:
- Keep constant tension on the ABs.
- Focus on feeling the AB muscles contract and move.
- Hold a total contraction when your knee meets your elbow.
- Don't let your shoulder and leg rest at the bottom of each repetition.
- Make sure you lower your elbow to the floor on each repetition.
- Make sure to keep your knee unlocked throughout movement.
- Keep small of back pressed against floor.

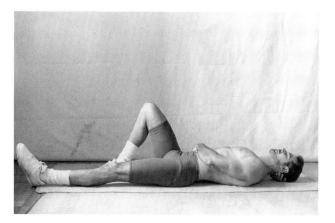

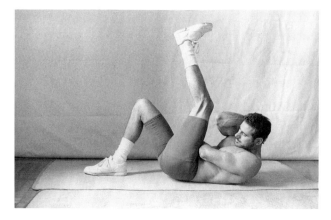

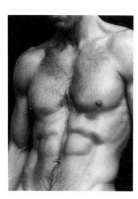

Exercise: Elbow to Knees: Double-Leg Cross

DIFFICULTY: 3
LOWER BACK: HIGH RISK
AREA: UPPER AND LOWER ABS
AND OBLIQUES

STARTING POSITION: Lie on your back. Extend your legs straight (knees unlocked). Raise your legs off the floor an inch and lean your upper body back to about a 45-degree angle.

MOVEMENT: Using your AB muscles, simultaneously bring both knees toward your left shoulder while curling the shoulder toward your knees. Lower body back to the starting position. Repeat to the opposite side.

Variation: Extend your legs straight (knees unlocked), heels on the floor. Execute the movement from this position.

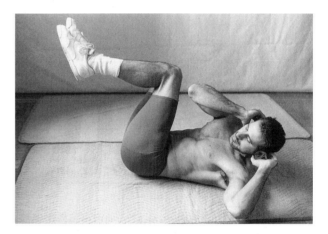

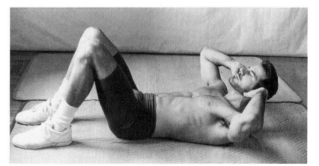

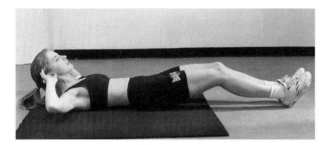

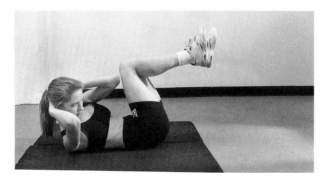

TRAINER'S TIPS:
- Concentrate on keeping constant tension on the ABs.
- Focus your mind on feeling your ABs do the work.
- Hold a total contraction at the top of the movement for a count of two.
- Don't let the leg touch the floor at the bottom of the movement.
- When returning to starting position, maintain a straight back—do not arc.

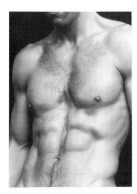

Exercise: Elbows to Knees: V Spread

DIFFICULTY: 2
LOWER BACK: HIGH RISK
AREA: UPPER AND LOWER ABS

STARTING POSITION: Lie flat on your back, knees bent, feet flat on the floor, head up (chin to chest), and hands behind your ears.

MOVEMENT: Use your ABs to simultaneously raise your legs and torso, bringing your elbows and knees together. As you lower your torso, shoot (spread or split) legs out, wide in a V position. From this position, bring your knees back together as you raise your torso, touching your knees to your elbows. This is all done in a fluid, continuous motion. Repeat.

TRAINER'S TIPS:
- Keep constant tension on the ABs.
- Don't let your legs touch the ground at any point in the movement.
- Focus on feeling your ABs moving the legs and the torso.
- Don't let the weight of your upper body rest on the floor during the exercise.
- Hold a total contraction for a count of two when the elbows and knees come together.
- Keep small of back pressed against ground.
- Spread and lower legs in a controlled motion. Keep the motion smooth.

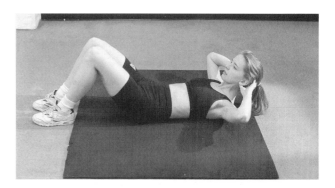

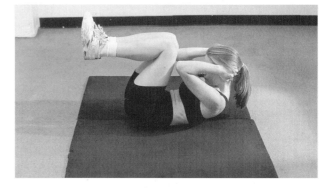

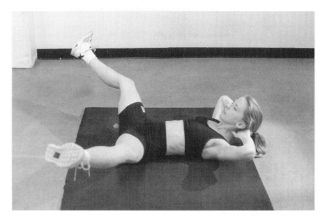

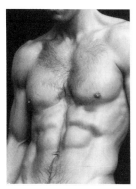

Exercise: Crunches with a Twist

DIFFICULTY: 2
LOWER BACK: MODERATE RISK
AREA: UPPER ABS AND OBLIQUES

STARTING POSITION: Lie flat on your back, knees up, feet flat on the floor, and hands in position of choice.

MOVEMENT: Use your AB muscles to twist your right shoulder toward your opposite knee in a forward-curling motion so your shoulder blades come off the mat. Repeat the movement to the opposite side.

Variations: You can incorporate this twisting movement (activating the oblique muscles) with all the Crunch variations (refer to Chapter 12 for photos of other variations): Frog Legs, Knees Up, Legs Straight, Legs Straight Up, Raised Hips, and on an incline board.

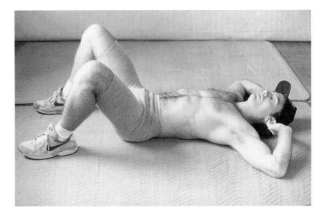

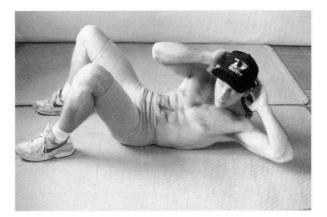

TRAINER'S TIPS:
- Hold a total contraction at the top of the movement for a count of two.
- Keep constant tension on the ABs. Don't rest at the bottom of the movement.
- Keep the movement isolated to your upper ABs and obliques. Don't come up too high.
- Focus your mind on feeling the ABs do the work.
- Remember this is a Crunch, so keep the small of your back pressed against the floor at all times.
- The top range of motion is complete when the nonworking shoulder blade comes slightly off the floor.
- On an incline board, increase the gradation as your strength increases.

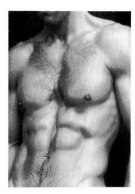

Exercise: Bench Crunches with a Cross

DIFFICULTY: 2
LOWER BACK: MODERATE RISK
AREA: UPPER ABS AND OBLIQUES

STARTING POSITION: Lie on your back on a bench, bending your knees, placing both feet flat on the bench. Then position your shoulder blades so they drop over the edge of the bench, and support your head with both hands.

MOVEMENT: Use your upper ABs to raise your torso as you twist your right shoulder toward your left knee. Then lower your shoulders below the bench and repeat.

TRAINER'S TIPS:
- Keep constant tension on your ABs throughout the full range of motion (both raising and lowering).
- Make sure you lower your shoulders below the bench on each repetition.
- Raise the torso as high as you would on a normal crunch.
- Don't rest at the bottom of the movement.
- Focus your mind on your upper ABs.

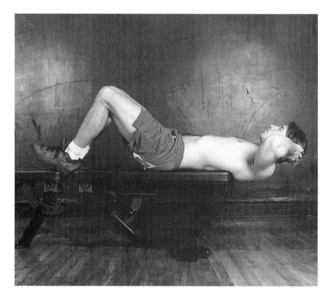

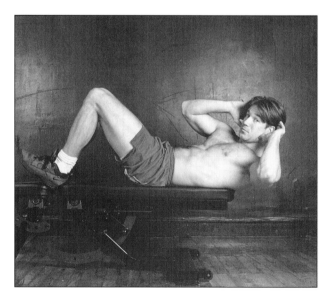

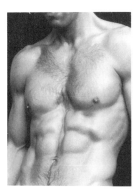

Exercise: Oblique Crunches

DIFFICULTY: 2
LOWER BACK: MODERATE RISK
AREA: UPPER AND LOWER ABS
AND OBLIQUES

STARTING POSITION: Lie flat on your back, letting both your legs fall to the left side so your right hip is perpendicular to your upper body. If your top leg won't go all the way down, let it rest in a comfortable position as close to the other leg as possible.

MOVEMENT: Keeping your shoulders as close to parallel to the floor as possible, use your AB muscles to raise both shoulder blades off the floor, bringing your rib cage toward your pelvis. Then lower your torso in a controlled motion. Repeat. Then switch sides.

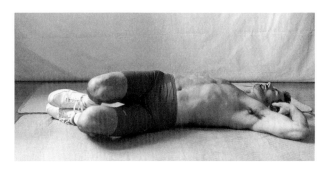

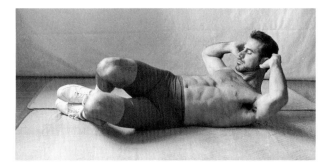

TRAINER'S TIPS:
- Focus your mind on feeling your ABs do the work.
- Keep constant tension on the ABs.
- Don't rest at the bottom of the movement.
- Make sure you move your shoulders off the floor. Don't just move your neck and head.
- Try not to lead the movement with a single shoulder. Keep the shoulders parallel to the floor.

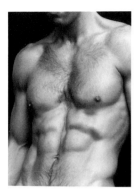

Exercise: Toe Touches with a Twist

DIFFICULTY: 2
LOWER BACK: MODERATE RISK
AREA: UPPER AND LOWER ABS
AND OBLIQUES

STARTING POSITION: Lie flat on your back, legs straight up (knees unlocked), perpendicular to your body, and arms extended toward ceiling.

MOVEMENT: Use your ABs to raise your right shoulder off the floor, touching the outside of your left ankle with your hand. Lower your shoulder back to the floor and repeat the movement to the opposite side, touching your left hand to the outside of your right ankle.

TRAINER'S TIPS:
- Concentrate on feeling the AB muscles do the work.
- Keep the movement controlled. Don't jerk up to reach the toes.
- Don't rest at the bottom of the movement. Keep tension on the ABs.
- If you can't touch your toes, just reach as far as you can. Your range of movement will improve with work.
- Keep small of back pressed against floor.

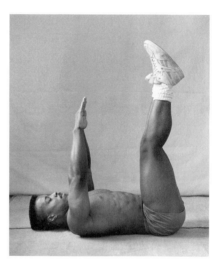

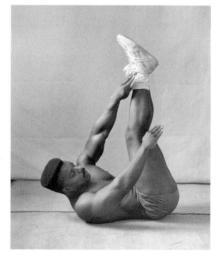

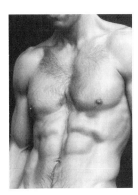

Exercise: Toe Touches: V Spread

DIFFICULTY: 2
LOWER BACK: LOW RISK
AREA: UPPER ABS AND OBLIQUES

STARTING POSITION: Lie on your back, legs straight up perpendicular to your body and spread in a V position (knees unlocked), and extend your arms toward the ceiling.

MOVEMENT: Use your AB muscles to raise both hands toward your left foot. Then lower your shoulder blades back down so they lightly touch the floor. Repeat to the opposite side.

TRAINER'S TIPS:

- Concentrate on feeling the AB muscles do the work.
- Don't reach up in a jerking motion. Keep it controlled.
- Don't rest at the bottom of the movement. When you feel your shoulders touch, start the next repetition.
- If you can't touch your toes, just reach as far as you can. Your range of movement will improve with work.
- If you have difficulty getting your legs to perpendicular, have a partner hold them or sit against a wall.
- Variation: Bring your legs as close to perpendicular as possible, reaching your hands straight up to the ceiling, instead of angling toward your toes.

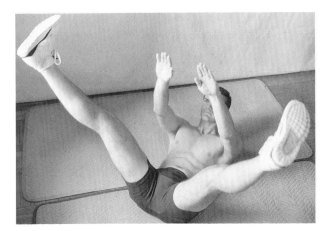

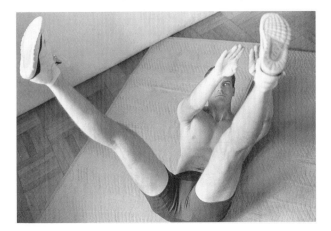

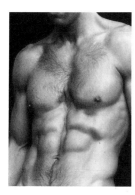

Exercise: Russian Twists

DIFFICULTY: 3
LOWER BACK: HIGH RISK
AREA: UPPER AND LOWER ABS
AND OBLIQUES

STARTING POSITION: Find a position of balance on your buttocks, feet in the air extended halfway out, hands clasped and extended out in front of you.

MOVEMENT: From this position. begin to twist side to side while maintaining balance on your buttocks, keeping constant tension on the ABs.

TRAINER'S TIPS:
- Don't crunch your body together. Keep good posture and try to relax into the position.
- Twist through a full range of motion, twisting as far to the right as you can then as far to your left as you can.
- Head and neck should remain lengthened and aligned with rest of spine.
- Don't move your head side to side.
- Maintain stable position on buttocks.

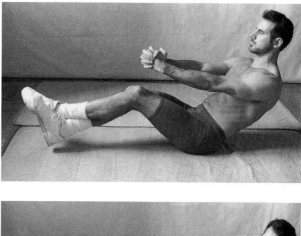

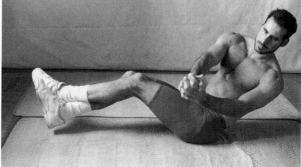

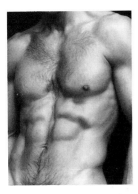

Exercise: Russian Twists: Roman Chair

DIFFICULTY: 2
LOWER BACK: HIGH RISK
AREA: UPPER AND LOWER ABS
AND OBLIQUES

STARTING POSITION: Sit on a Roman chair, put your feet under the support handles, and lean back to about a 45-degree angle, so you feel tension on your upper and lower ABs. Extend your hands out in front of you and clasp them together. You can also do this exercise holding a broom handle or a light pole across the back of your shoulders.

MOVEMENT: From this position, twist to your right, then back to your left, while keeping constant tension on the ABs.

TRAINER'S TIPS:
- Lean back about midway between being parallel to the floor and sitting straight up.
- Don't crunch your body together—lengthen it and relax.
- Go through a full range of motion—twist as far to your right as you can, and then twist as far to your left as you can.
- Don't move your head side to side.

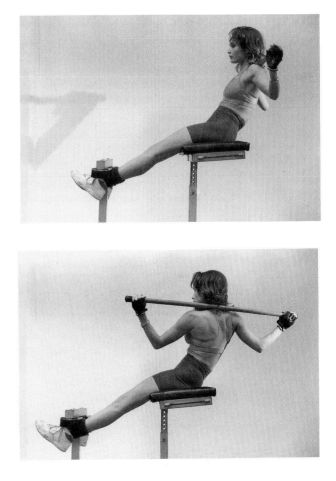

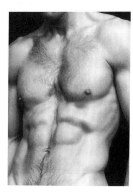

Exercise: Navratilova Twists

DIFFICULTY: 2
LOWER BACK: HIGH RISK
AREA: UPPER AND LOWER ABS
AND OBLIQUES

STARTING POSITION: Sit on a Roman chair, put your feet under the support handles, and lean back to about a 45-degree angle, so you feel tension on your upper and lower ABs. Place your hands behind your ears or hold a broom handle or a light pole across the back of your shoulders.

MOVEMENT: Use your ABs to cross your torso diagonally toward your opposite leg. Return to the starting position and repeat to the opposite side.

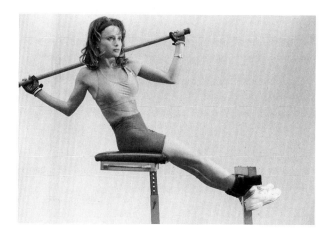

TRAINER'S TIPS:
- Don't twist your torso—angle it.
- The motion is similar to the crossing motion in a serve.
- Lean back about midway between being parallel to the floor and sitting straight up.
- Don't crunch your body together—lengthen it and relax.

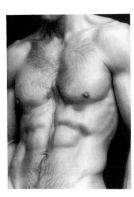

Exercise: Oblique Crosses: V Spread (Legs Down)

DIFFICULTY: 2
LOWER BACK: MODERATE RISK
AREA: UPPER AND LOWER ABS AND OBLIQUES

STARTING POSITION: Lie flat on your back, legs fully extended on the floor and spread in a V position (knees unlocked) and hands in position of choice.

MOVEMENT: Use the muscles of your ABs to raise your torso over your left leg. Go up as high as you can while keeping your lower back pressed against the floor. Then lower your body in a controlled motion. Repeat to the opposite side.

TRAINER'S TIPS:
- Make sure your torso crosses toward your leg, activating the obliques.
- Keep constant tension on the ABs.
- Don't rest on the floor after lowering your shoulders down.
- Focus your mind on feeling your ABs do the work.
- Keep small of back pressed against floor.

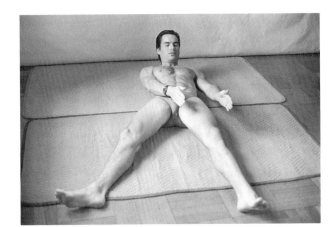

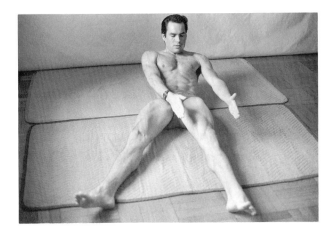

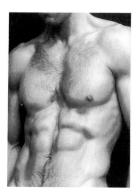

Exercise: Oblique Crosses: V Spread (Leg Up)

DIFFICULTY: 2
LOWER BACK: HIGH RISK
AREA: UPPER AND LOWER ABS
AND OBLIQUES

STARTING POSITION: Lie flat on your back, legs fully extended and spread in a V position (knees unlocked) and hands in position of choice.

MOVEMENT: Lift your left leg off the floor about twelve inches. Then use your AB muscles to raise your torso over your raised leg. Go up as high as you can while keeping your lower back pressed against the floor. The leg stays at the same level. Then lower your body in a controlled motion. Then repeat the exercise on the opposite leg.

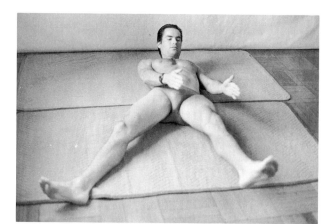

TRAINER'S TIPS:
- Make sure you cross your torso toward the leg, contracting the obliques.
- Keep constant tension on the ABs.
- Don't rest on the floor after lowering your shoulders down.
- Focus your mind on feeling your ABs do the work.
- Don't let the raised leg touch the floor during the set.
- Keep small of back pressed to floor.

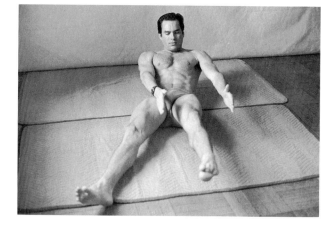

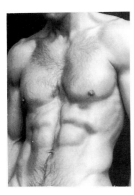

Exercise: Knee-ups

DIFFICULTY: 2
LOWER BACK: MODERATE RISK
AREA: LOWER AND UPPER ABS

STARTING POSITION: Sit on a bench, holding on to the side for support. Extend your legs straight, keeping a slight bend in the knees. Raise your legs off the floor an inch and lean the upper body back to about a 45-degree angle.

Variation (On the Floor): Sit on the floor, lifting your legs off the floor and balancing on your buttocks. Then place your hands behind your hips for support.

MOVEMENT: Use your ABs to lift your knees toward your chest while simultaneously raising your upper body toward your knees. Then simultaneously return upper body and lower body back to the starting position.

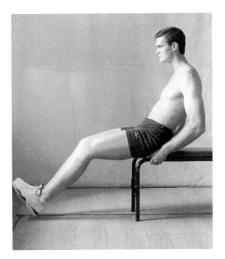

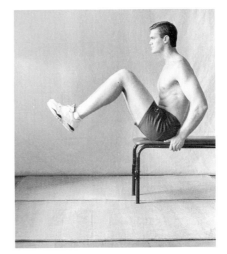

TRAINER'S TIPS:
- Concentrate on keeping constant tension on the AB muscles.
- Focus your mind on feeling the ABs do the work, not the legs and hip flexors.
- When the knees and ABs come together, hold a total contraction for a count of two.
- Don't let the legs touch the floor at the bottom of the movement.
- Keep back straight when returning to starting position.

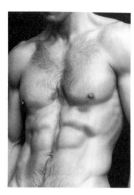

Exercise: Knee-ups: Double-Leg Cross

DIFFICULTY: 3
LOWER BACK: HIGH RISK
AREA: UPPER AND LOWER ABS
AND OBLIQUES

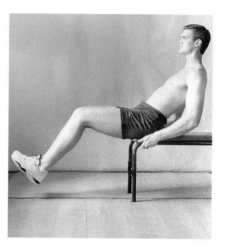

STARTING POSITION: Sit on a bench holding on to the back side for support. Extend your legs straight (knees unlocked). Raise your legs off the floor an inch and lean your upper body back to about a 45-degree angle.

MOVEMENT: Using your AB muscles, simultaneously bring both knees toward your left shoulder, while curling the shoulder toward your knees. Lower body back to the starting position. Repeat to the opposite side.

TRAINER'S TIPS:
- Concentrate on keeping constant tension on the ABs.
- Focus your mind on feeling your ABs do the work.
- Hold a total contraction at the top of the movement for a count of two.
- Don't let the leg touch the floor at the bottom of the movement.
- When returning to starting position, maintain a straight back. Do not arch.

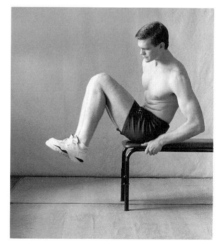

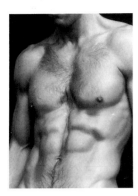

Exercise: Leg Scissors Crunches

DIFFICULTY: 3
LOWER BACK: HIGH RISK
AREA: UPPER ABS AND LOWER ABS

STARTING POSITION: Lie flat on your back, legs fully extended (knees unlocked), heels resting on the floor, and hands behind your head.

MOVEMENT: Use your ABs to raise your shoulder blades off the floor as you simultaneously raise your left leg as close to perpendicular to the floor as you can. Then simultaneously lower your leg and torso. Repeat with right leg and torso.

TRAINER'S TIPS:
- Think of raising your leg a split second before your torso.
- Keep constant tension on your ABs throughout the full range of motion (all directions).
- Raise your torso as high as you would on a normal crunch.
- Don't rest at the bottom of the movement.
- Keep your legs straight (but knees unlocked).
- Focus your mind on your ABs.

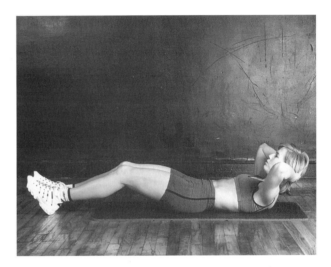

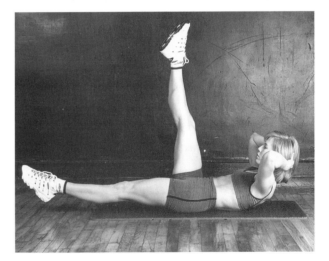

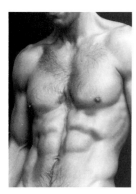

Exercise: Leg Scissors Crunches with a Cross

DIFFICULTY: 3

LOWER BACK: HIGH RISK

AREA: UPPER ABS, OBLIQUES, AND LOWER ABS

STARTING POSITION: Lie flat on your back, legs fully extended (knees unlocked), heels resting on the floor, and hands behind your head.

MOVEMENT: Use your ABs to raise and cross your right shoulder toward your left leg, as you simultaneously raise the left leg (bring leg as close to perpendicular as possible). Then simultaneously lower your leg and torso. Repeat cross with left shoulder.

TRAINER'S TIPS:
- Think of raising your leg a split second before your torso.
- Keep constant tension on your ABs throughout the full range of motion (all directions).
- Raise your torso as high as you would on a normal crunch.
- Don't rest at the bottom of the movement.
- Keep your legs straight (but knees unlocked).
- Focus your mind on your ABs.

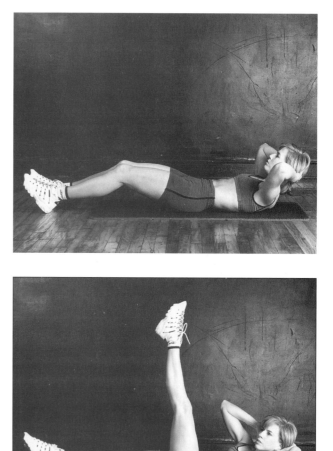

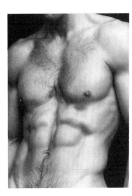

Exercise: V-ups

DIFFICULTY: 3
LOWER BACK: HIGH RISK
AREA: UPPER AND LOWER ABS

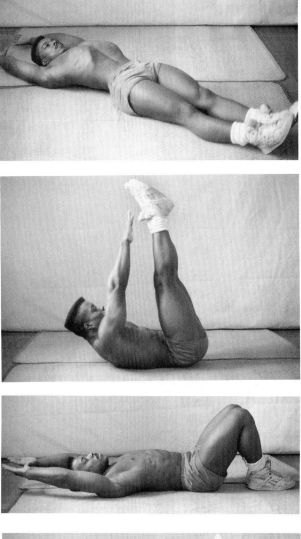

STARTING POSITION: Lie flat on your back, legs extended straight (knees unlocked), heels resting on floor, arms extended overhead.

MOVEMENT: Use ABs to simultaneously raise your torso and legs together so your hands touch your feet, and your legs and arms are pointing up in a closed V. Then, in a controlled motion, lower your legs and torso back to the starting position. Repeat.

Bent-Knee Variation: Same starting position, except you have your knees bent and feet flat on the ground. The movement is the same, except you keep your knees bent throughout the range of motion, and you end each repetition in the bent-knee position.

TRAINER'S TIPS:
- Focus on feeling your AB muscles pull your torso and legs together.
- Keep the movement controlled—don't jerk yourself up.
- Don't rest your arms and legs at the bottom of the movement.
- Hold a total contraction at the top of the movement for a count of two.
- Focus your mind on feeling your ABs do the work.
- The bent-knee version is easier and puts less stress on your back.

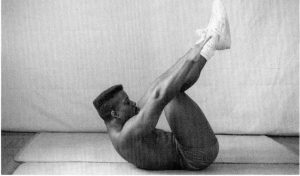

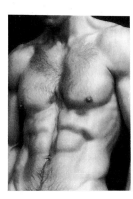

Exercise: V-ups with a Cross

DIFFICULTY: 3
LOWER BACK: HIGH RISK
**AREA: UPPER ABS, OBLIQUES,
AND LOWER ABS**

STARTING POSITION: Lie flat on your back, legs fully extended (knees unlocked), heels resting on the floor, and arms extended over head.

MOVEMENT: Use your ABs to simultaneously bring your feet and hands together. As you raise your torso and legs, cross your right shoulder toward your left knee and your left knee toward your right shoulder. Then simultaneously lower your leg and torso.

TRAINER'S TIPS:
- Think of raising your legs a split second before your torso.
- Keep constant tension on your ABs throughout the full range of motion (all directions).
- Don't rest at the bottom of the movement.
- Keep your legs straight (but don't lock your knees).
- Focus your mind on your ABs.

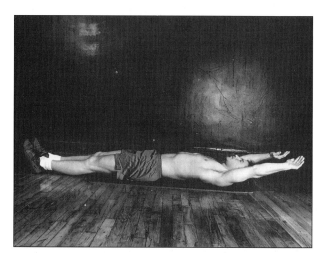

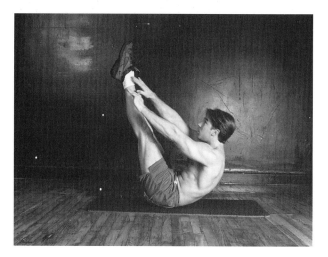

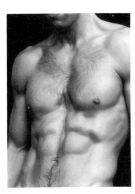

Exercise: Side Knee-ups

DIFFICULTY: 2
LOWER BACK: MODERATE RISK
AREA: OBLIQUES, LOWER AND UPPER ABS

STARTING POSITION: Lie on your left buttock, legs fully extended (knees unlocked), left arm out front for support, and right hand behind your ear.

MOVEMENT: Use your ABs to simultaneously raise your legs and torso off the floor, bringing your knees and chest together. Then return to the starting position. Repeat. Complete your set, then switch sides.

TRAINER'S TIPS:
- Don't let your legs and torso rest on the floor at the bottom of the movement.
- Hold a total contraction at the top of the movement for a count of two.
- Focus your mind on feeling your ABs do the work.

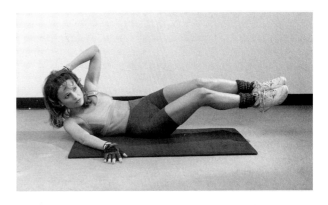

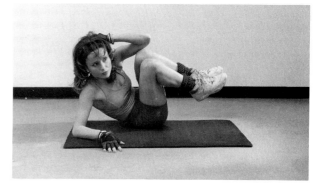

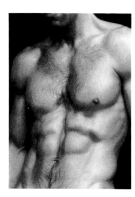

Exercise: Full Sit-ups: Bent Knee

DIFFICULTY: 3
LOWER BACK: HIGH RISK
AREA: UPPER AND LOWER ABS

STARTING POSITION: Lie on your back, knees bent, feet flat on the floor, and hands in position of choice.

MOVEMENT: Use your ABs to roll your spine up to a sitting position. Then, without resting at the top of the movement, lower yourself back to the starting position. Repeat.

Incline Board Variation: Follow the same instructions as above.

TRAINER'S TIPS:
- Keep the movement fluid and controlled.
- Don't bounce at the bottom or jerk your chest and shoulders upward to get momentum.
- Keep constant tension on the stomach during both the raising and lowering phases.
- Focus your mind on feeling your ABs do the work.
- Keep your feet flat on the floor.
- Keep lower back slightly rounded through both ranges of motion.
- Hold a total contraction at the top of the movement for a count of two.

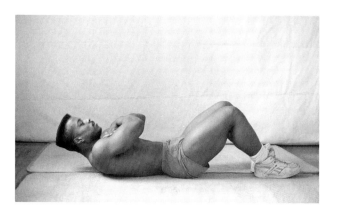

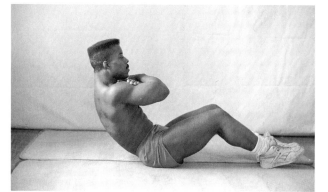

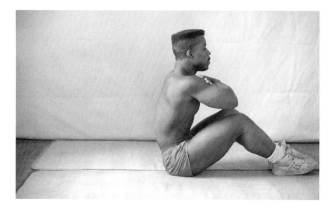

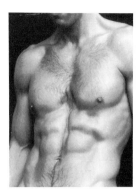

Exercise: Full Sit-ups with a Twist

DIFFICULTY: 3
LOWER BACK: HIGH RISK
AREA: UPPER AND LOWER ABS

STARTING POSITION: Lie flat on your back, knees bent, feet flat on the floor, and hands in position of choice.

MOVEMENT: Use your ABs to roll your spine off the floor to a sitting position; as the small of your back comes off the floor, twist your right shoulder toward your opposite knee. Lower your torso back to the starting position, and repeat to the opposite side.

TRAINER'S TIPS:
- Keep the movement fluid and controlled.
- Don't jerk or bounce at the bottom to help yourself up.
- Hold a total contraction at the top of the movement for a count of two.
- Keep constant tension on the stomach during both the raising and lowering phases.
- Keep lower back slightly rounded through both ranges of motion.

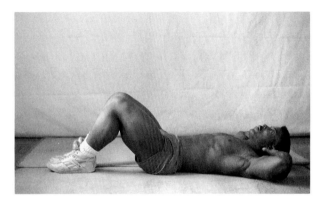

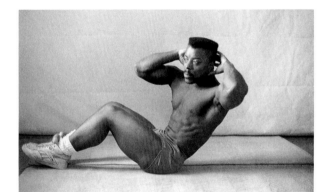

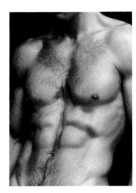

Exercise: Full Sit-ups: Feet Up

DIFFICULTY: 3
LOWER BACK: HIGH RISK
AREA: UPPER AND LOWER ABS

STARTING POSITION: Lie flat on your back, thighs perpendicular to your body, knees together, feet extended parallel to the floor, and hands in position of choice. It is helpful to rest your lower legs over something: an exercise bench or a chair.

MOVEMENT: Use ABs to roll your spine up, bringing your forehead as close to your knees as possible. If you can't make it that high, your range of motion will improve with work. Repeat.

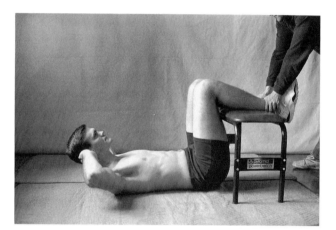

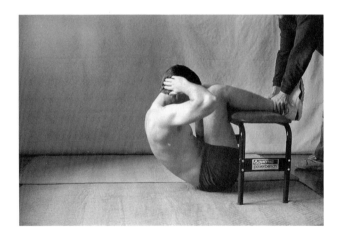

TRAINER'S TIPS:
- Don't bounce or jerk at the bottom of the movement.
- Keep constant tension on the ABs throughout the entire range of motion.
- Don't let yourself just fall back to the floor—keep the contraction through both the raising and lowering phases.
- Hold a total contraction at the top of the movement for a count of two.
- It is helpful to have someone hold your ankles during this movement.
- Keep your knees together throughout the movement.
- Keep your hips directly under your knees throughout the movement.
- Keep lower back slightly rounded through both ranges of motion.

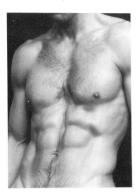

Exercise: Full Sit-ups: Feet Up and Twist

DIFFICULTY: 3
LOWER BACK: HIGH RISK
AREA: UPPER AND LOWER ABS
AND OBLIQUES

STARTING POSITION: Lie flat on your back, thighs perpendicular to your body, knees together, feet extended parallel to the floor, and hands in position of choice. It is helpful to rest your lower legs over something—an exercise bench or a chair.

MOVEMENT: Use ABs to roll your spine up, as you twist your right shoulder toward your opposite knee, bringing your shoulder as close to your knee as possible. If you can't make it that far, your range of motion will improve with work. Repeat.

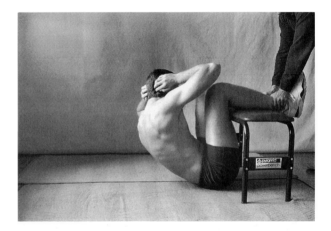

TRAINER'S TIPS:
- Don't bounce or jerk at the bottom of the movement.
- Keep constant tension on the stomach throughout the entire range of motion.
- Don't just let yourself fall back to the floor—keep the contraction through both the raising and lowering phases.
- Hold a total contraction at the top of the movement for a count of two.
- It is helpful to have someone hold your ankles during this movement.
- Keep your knees together throughout the movement.
- Keep your hips directly under your knees throughout the movement.
- Keep lower back slightly rounded through both ranges of motion.

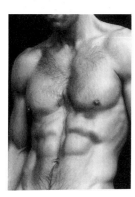

Exercise: Roman Chair Sit-ups

DIFFICULTY: 2
LOWER BACK: HIGH RISK
AREA: UPPER AND LOWER ABS

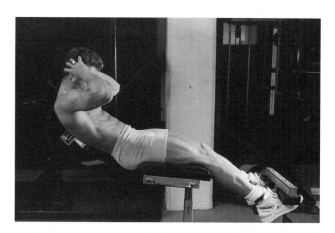

STARTING POSITION: Sit on the Roman Chair—put your feet under the support handles and hands in position of choice. Lower the support handles to a level that stabilizes you throughout the entire movement.

MOVEMENT: Rounding your back, use your ABs to lower your torso as close to parallel to the floor as possible. Then raise your body back to the starting position. Repeat.

Variation: This movement can also be done with a twist.

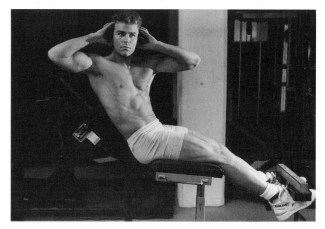

TRAINER'S TIPS:
- Keep the movement fluid and controlled.
- Don't bounce at the bottom or jerk your chest and shoulders upward to get momentum.
- Keep constant tension on the stomach during both the raising and lowering phases.
- Focus your mind on feeling your ABs do the work.
- Hold a total contraction at the top of the movement for a count of two.

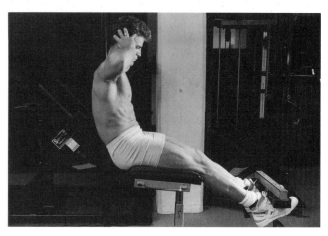

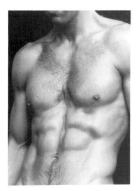

Exercise: Sit-ups: Negative

DIFFICULTY: 2
LOWER BACK: HIGH RISK
AREA: UPPER ABS

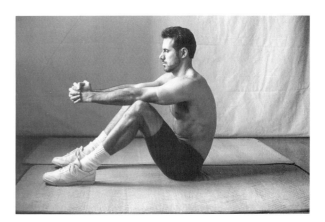

STARTING POSITION: Sit, knees bent, chest against your thighs. feet flat on the floor, arms extended in front, and hands clasped.

MOVEMENT: Lower yourself back, curling your torso forward and rounding your lower back. Continue to lower your torso until your upper ABs feel locked. Then raise yourself to the sitting position.*

Variation: This exercise can also be done on an incline board.

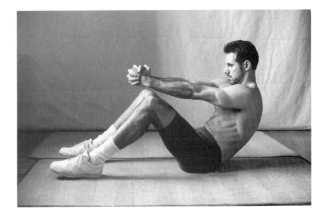

TRAINER'S TIPS:
• As you lower yourself, keep the small of your back rounded.
• One sign that the upper ABs are in position to lock is the feeling that to go down any farther would shift the tension off your ABs and put the pressure on your lower back.
• When returning to the sitting position, only go high enough to keep tension on the ABs. When you feel tension go off the ABs, you've gone up too far.
• Concentrate on feeling your AB muscles do the work.
• At the bottom of the movement, hold a total contraction for a count of two.
• The farther you move your heels from your buttocks, the more emphasis you'll put on your lower ABs.

* If you have a bad lower back, proceed with caution. Make sure you keep the back rounded and contracted for support, and be careful not to lower yourself too far.

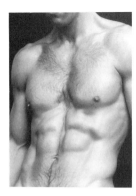

Exercise: Body Tuck

DIFFICULTY: 3
LOWER BACK: HIGH RISK
AREA: UPPER AND LOWER ABS

STARTING POSITION: Lie flat on your back, legs fully extended (knees unlocked), and hands in position of choice.

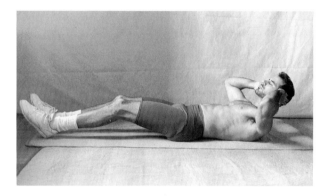

MOVEMENT: Raise your entire torso off the floor by rolling your spine to a sitting position, while simultaneously bringing your heels toward your buttocks until you are in a tucked sitting position. Then lower your torso and extend your legs back to the starting position.

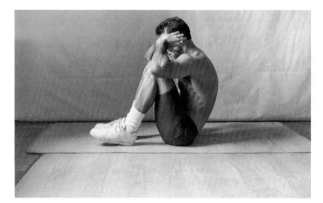

TRAINER'S TIPS:
- This exercise should be done in a slow, controlled motion.
- Hold a total contraction at the top of the movement.
- Don't rest at the conclusion of the movement— start your next repetition.
- Focus on feeling your AB muscles moving your legs and upper body.
- Keep your knees unlocked when your legs are fully extended.
- Keep your lower back pressed against the floor for as much of the movement as possible.
- Drag your heels across the floor toward your buttocks as you bring your knees up.
- Keep lower back slightly rounded through both ranges of motion.

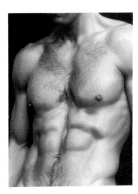

Exercise: Body Tuck: Half Sit-up

DIFFICULTY: 2
LOWER BACK: MODERATE RISK
AREA: UPPER AND LOWER ABS

STARTING POSITION: Lie flat on your back, legs fully extended (knees unlocked), and hands in position of choice.

MOVEMENT: Use your ABs to raise your torso so your shoulder blades come off the floor, while simultaneously bringing your heels to your buttocks. Then lower your torso and extend your legs back to the starting position. Repeat.

Twist Variation: This exercise can also be done with a twist. As you raise your torso, cross your right shoulder toward your left knee. Repeat to the other side.

TRAINER'S TIPS:
- This exercise should be done in a slow, controlled motion.
- Hold a total contraction for a count of two at the top of the movement.
- Don't rest at the conclusion of the movement—start your next repetition.
- Focus on feeling your AB muscles moving your legs and upper body.
- Keep your lower back pressed against the floor.
- Drag your heels across the floor when bringing your knees up.

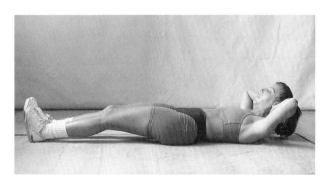

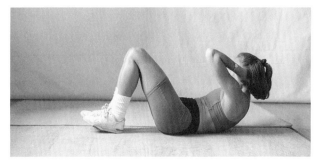

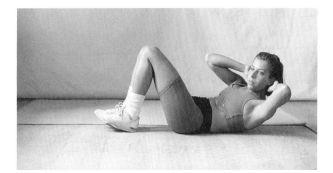

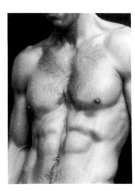

Exercise: Hanging Leg Raises with a Cross: Both Legs

DIFFICULTY: 2
LOWER BACK: MODERATE RISK
AREA: UPPER AND LOWER ABS
AND OBLIQUES

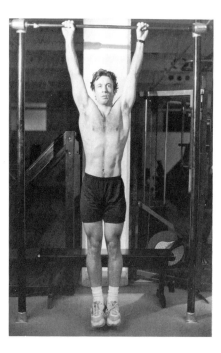

STARTING POSITION: Hang from a bar or vertical chair with your legs fully extended and hands a little wider than shoulder width.

MOVEMENT: Use your ABs to cross and raise both legs (knees unlocked) to the outside of your left hand. Then lower them back to the starting position. Repeat the movement to the opposite side, raising your legs to the outside of your right hand.

TRAINER'S TIPS:

- Don't let your legs rest at the bottom of the movement.
- Hold a total contraction at the top of the movement.
- Let your hips move forward as your leg passes the 90-degree angle.
- Don't swing to gain momentum.
- Control the motion on the way down. Don't just let your legs drop.
- Focus your mind on feeling the ABs do the work.
- If you can't get your feet all the way up, just go as high as you can. Your range of motion will improve with work.
- The nonworking leg will move slightly forward as the crossing leg reaches the top of the movement.

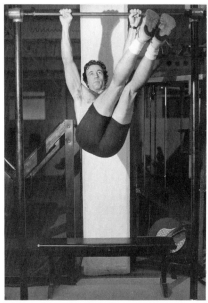

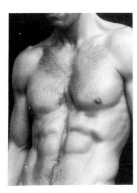

Exercise: Hanging Leg Raises with a Cross: Straight Leg

DIFFICULTY: 3
LOWER BACK: MODERATE RISK
AREA: UPPER AND LOWER ABS AND OBLIQUES

STARTING POSITION: Hang from a bar or vertical chair with your legs fully extended and hands slightly wider than shoulder width apart.

MOVEMENT: Use your ABs to raise and cross your right leg (knee unlocked) to the outside of your left hand. Then lower your leg in a controlled motion back to the starting position. Repeat the movement to the opposite side, bringing your left foot to the outside of your right hand.

TRAINER'S TIPS:
- Don't rest at the bottom of the movement.
- Hold a total contraction at the top of the movement.
- Let your hips move forward as your legs pass the 90-degree angle.
- Don't swing to gain momentum.
- Control the motion on the way down. Don't just let your leg drop.
- Focus your mind on feeling the ABs do the work.
- If you can't get your feet all the way up, just go as high as you can. Your range of motion will improve with work.

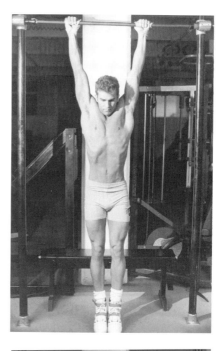

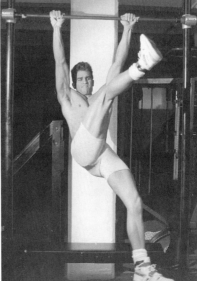

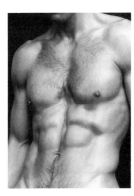

Exercise: Hanging Knee Raises with a Cross

DIFFICULTY: 3
LOWER BACK: MODERATE RISK
AREA: UPPER AND LOWER ABS
AND OBLIQUES

STARTING POSITION: Hang from a bar or vertical chair, legs fully extended and hands a little wider than shoulder width.

MOVEMENT: Use your AB muscles to raise your knees in a crossing motion toward your left shoulder. Then lower them back to the starting position. Repeat the movement to the opposite side.

TRAINER'S TIPS:
- Don't let your legs rest at the bottom of the movement.
- Hold a total contraction at the top of the movement.
- Let your hips move forward as your knees pass the 90-degree angle.
- Don't swing to gain momentum.
- Control the motion on the way down. Don't just let your legs drop.
- Focus your mind on feeling the ABs do the work.
- If you can't get your knees all the way up, just go as high as you can. Your range of motion will improve with work.

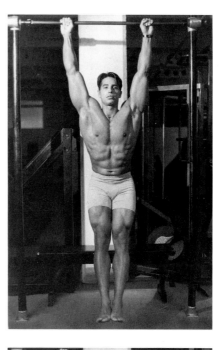

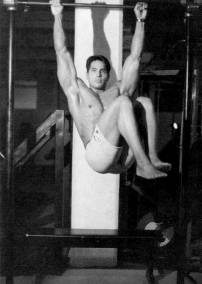

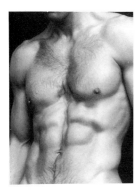

Exercise: Hanging Knee Raises with a Cross: Single Knee

DIFFICULTY: 2
LOWER BACK: MODERATE RISK
**AREA: UPPER AND LOWER ABS
AND OBLIQUES**

STARTING POSITION: Hang from a bar or vertical chair with your feet fully extended and hands a little wider than shoulder width.

MOVEMENT: Use your ABs to cross your right knee toward your left shoulder. Then lower it back to the starting position. Repeat the movement to the opposite side. Cross your left knee to your right shoulder.

TRAINER'S TIPS:
- Don't let your leg rest at the bottom of the movement.
- Hold a total contraction at the top of the movement.
- Let your hips move forward as your knees pass the 90-degree angle.
- Don't swing to gain momentum.
- Control the motion on the way down. Don't just let your leg drop.
- Focus your mind on feeling the ABs do the work.

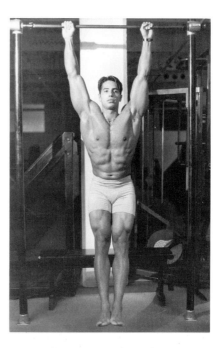

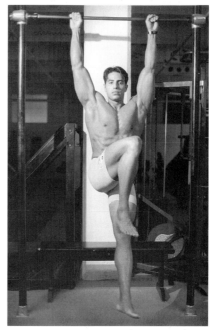

THE COMPLETE BOOK OF ABS

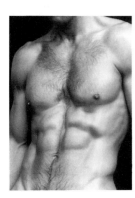

Exercise: Cable Crunches with a Cross

DIFFICULTY: 3
LOWER BACK: LOW RISK
AREA: UPPER ABS AND OBLIQUES

STARTING POSITION: Grab the cable attachment. Kneel facing the machine, hips off your heels, holding the attachment, with both hands, at your forehead.

MOVEMENT: Using the muscles of your ABs, bend over and forward, driving your right shoulder toward your opposite knee, while keeping the cable tight and held stationary to your forehead. Raise your torso up to about a 45-degree angle. Then bend forward, crossing your left shoulder over your right knee. Repeat to the opposite side.

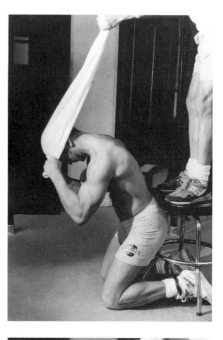

TRAINER'S TIPS:
- Raise and lower the weights in a controlled motion. Don't pop up.
- Don't come all the way up on each repetition—maintain approximately the 45-degree angle.
- Hold a total contraction for a count of two at the bottom of the movement.
- Focus your mind on feeling your ABs do the work.

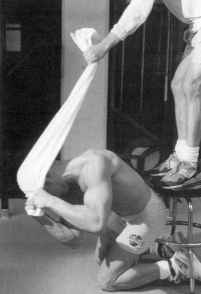

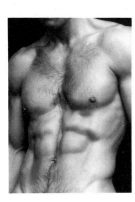

Exercise: Pelvic Tilts

DIFFICULTY: 1
LOWER BACK: LOW RISK
AREA: UPPER AND LOWER ABS

STARTING POSITION: Lie flat on your back, knees bent, feet flat, hands in position of choice.

MOVEMENT: Rotate your pelvis up and toward your rib cage, pushing the small of your back against the floor. Then let the pelvis rotate back to its normal position so that the lower back comes off the ground.

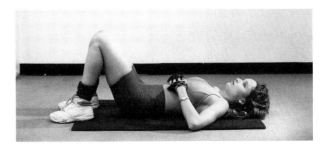

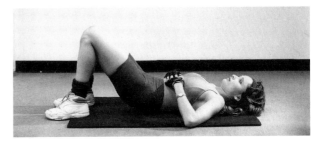

TRAINER'S TIPS:
- Don't lift your buttocks off the floor instead of rotating the hips.
- This is a subtle movement. You are using your stomach muscles to rotate the pelvis toward your rib cage to put it in a tilt.
- This is an important position to understand, because placing yourself in this position can help prevent lower-back strain.
- When you are in the tilt position, hold an isometric contraction for a count of two.

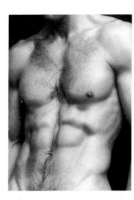

Exercise: Vacuums

DIFFICULTY: 2
LOWER BACK: LOW RISK
AREA: TRANSVERSE ABDOMINIS

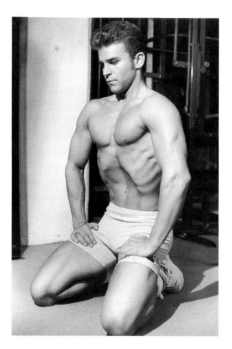

STARTING POSITION: 1) On all fours. 2) Kneeling, hands on thighs, heels on buttocks, back straight. 3) Standing, legs slightly bent, hands on thighs.

MOVEMENT: Exhale all the air from your body, and suck your abdomen up and in as far as you can. Hold for 10 seconds. Relax and repeat.

TRAINER'S TIPS:
- Focus on pulling the ABs up and in.
- Each starting position will get progressively harder, all fours being the easiest and standing the hardest.
- Start out holding each exhalation for 10 seconds, and gradually work up to 30 seconds.

CHAPTER FOURTEEN

Isometrics

Introduction to Isometrics

The concept of isometric training is not new. It has been popular since the days of Charles Atlas. He promised to turn a ninety-eight-pound weakling (who got sand kicked in his face) into a muscle man who gets the girl.

Isometrics fell out of popularity for a number of years, but as with many concepts in fitness, it is again becoming popular. Some of the reasons are: the ease of technique, new findings about strength gains through a greater range of motion, and the value of variation in your workouts.

This chapter will provide you with isometric abdominal exercises for your ABs, and hopefully inspire you to create your own variations. The exercises that you will encounter in this chapter are specific isometric exercises, but you are limited only by your imagination in the application of these techniques. You can apply isometrics to any exercise you perform.

Isometrics Defined

Isometric means "same length." An isometric contraction occurs when a muscle gains tension but does not change in length. Isometrics involve no joint movement, but permit maximum muscular contraction. The strength development is specific to only one angle rather than through a full range of motion. Although tension does develop, no mechanical work is performed. Also referred to as "static" contractions, the technique of an isometric hold is simply to contract the muscle, squeeze it tight, and hold the contraction for the prescribed amount of time.

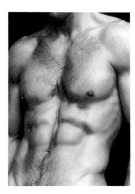

Exercise: Isometric Seated Leg Raises

DIFFICULTY: 1
LOWER BACK: LOW RISK
AREA: LOWER ABS

STARTING POSITION: Seated on a chair or bench, place your hands on your thighs just above your knees and lean your torso slightly back. Then lift your feet off the floor a couple of inches.

THE SQUEEZE: Use your lower ABs to press your thighs up against your hands. Don't let your thighs move more than an inch or so off the chair. Hold the static position ten seconds and relax. Repeat.

MOVEMENT VARIATION 1: The same as above, but lift one leg at a time.

MOVEMENT VARIATION 2: Hook your feet under an immovable resistance, such as a desk or the airplane seat in front of you. Then attempt to bring your knees to your chest. Use your arms to hang onto the armrests or the sides of the chair for support.

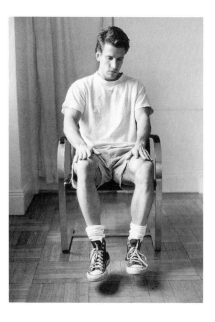

TRAINER'S TIPS:
- Feel the tension in the abdominals.
- Maintain regular breathing during ten-second contractions.
- Visualize bringing your knees to your chest.
- Focus your mind on feeling your ABs do the work.
- Keep your lower back rounded during the contraction.
- Contract your ABs as tightly as possible during the hold.

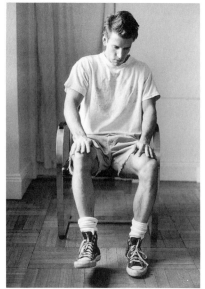

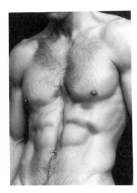

Exercise: Isometric Cross Pushes

DIFFICULTY: 1
LOWER BACK: LOW RISK
AREA: LOWER ABS AND OBLIQUES

STARTING POSITION: Sit in a chair, lean torso slightly back, place your right hand on your left thigh just above the knee and bring your foot an inch off the floor.

THE SQUEEZE: Use your ABs to attempt to raise your knee toward your opposite shoulder and lower your shoulder toward your opposite knee, blocking movement with your right hand. Hold for ten seconds and relax. Repeat the movement on the other side.

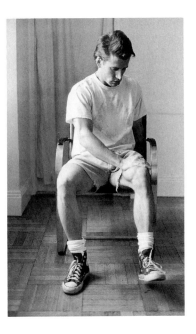

TRAINER'S TIPS:
- Feel the tension in the ABs.
- Maintain regular breathing during ten-second contractions.
- Concentrate on moving knee to opposing shoulder and shoulder to opposing knee.
- Don't allow the foot to come off the floor more than a couple of inches.
- Focus your mind on feeling your ABs do the work.

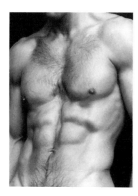

Exercise: Isometric Oblique Bends

DIFFICULTY: 1
LOWER BACK: LOW RISK
AREA: OBLIQUES

STARTING POSITION: Stand three to six inches from a wall or post, leaning the outside of your shoulder against it, feet parallel to the wall, with your arms folded across your chest.

THE SQUEEZE: Use your oblique muscles to push your shoulder into the wall or post. Hold contraction for ten seconds and then relax. Repeat the movement on the other side.

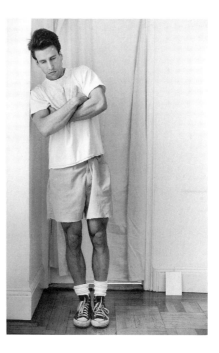

TRAINER'S TIPS:
- Do not twist your torso.
- Feel the tension in the obliques.
- Visualize driving your shoulder through the wall.
- Maintain regular breathing during ten-second contractions.
- You can vary the exercise by moving closer or farther from the wall.
- Make sure you are pushing with your oblique muscles, not your legs.
- Focus your mind on feeling your ABs do the work.

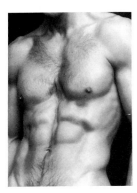

Exercise: Isometric AB Pushdowns

DIFFICULTY: 1
LOWER BACK: LOW RISK
AREA: UPPER ABS

STARTING POSITION: Sit in a chair, place your hands on your thighs (just above your knees), fingers facing in toward each other and torso bent forward at approximately a 45-degree angle.

THE SQUEEZE: Contract your ABs as you attempt to push your chest toward your thighs—let your arms block the movement as you maintain the 45-degree angle. Hold contraction for ten seconds. Repeat.

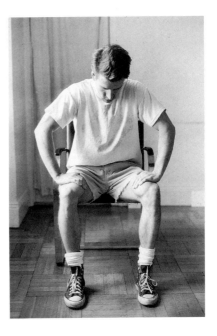

TRAINER'S TIPS:
- Feel the tension in the ABs.
- Maintain regular breathing during ten-second contractions.
- Imagine you are trying to push your hands through your thighs.
- Focus your mind on feeling your ABs do the work.
- Contract your ABs as tightly as possible during the hold.

CHAPTER FIFTEEN

The Machines

by DAVE JOHNSON

Machine Introduction

The purpose of this chapter is to serve as a resource: to outline some of the popular machines found in health clubs, and to give you instructional guidelines. Sometimes it is hard to receive personal instruction at a gym. The manufacturer's instructions and illustrations found in this chapter will give you the opportunity to review at home proper machine usage. As with any of the other AB exercises, it is extremely important to master the technique of using the machines in order to ensure safety and to gain optimum results. It is best to get qualified instruction from a trainer at your club about proper usage. Don't be shy about asking. That's his or her job.

As you will see, most of the machines use crunchlike movements for the rectus abdominis and twisting movements for the obliques. A couple of the machines are designed to work the lower ABs. Using the machines along with doing other exercises can enhance your AB workout.

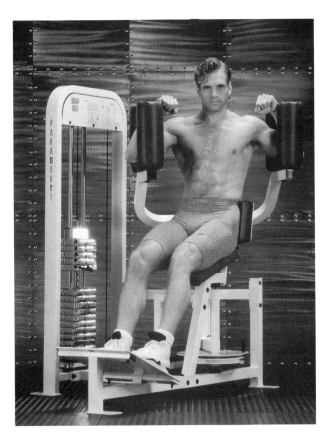

Paramount—Rotary Torso

A. INSTRUCTIONS

1. Set weight resistance desired.

2. Adjust seat and place feet in platforms.

3. Adjust range-of-motion limiter to desired position.

4. Exercise turning left and holding. Then turn back to start position. Do the same for the opposite side.

B. MUSCLES TRAINED

1. Internal obliques

2. External obliques

Paramount—Abdominal

A. INSTRUCTIONS

1. From a seated position, select desired weight amount.

2. Adjust seat so that pivot point aligns with the mid-torso.

3. Place feet under the forward or rear roller pads.

4. Grasp the foam handles and lean forward.

5. Return to initial position and repeat.

B. MUSCLES TRAINED

1. Rectus abdominis

2. Iliopsoas group

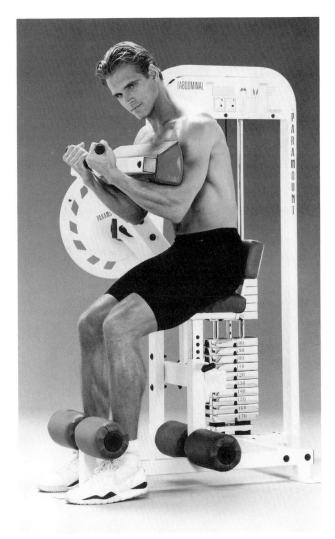

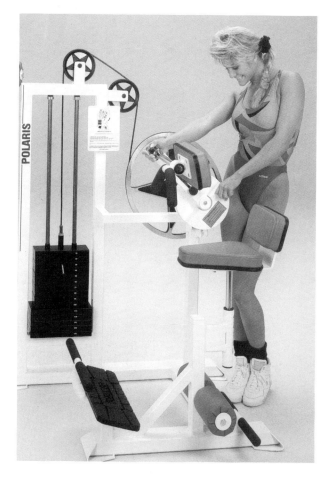

Polaris—Abdominal

A. INSTRUCTIONS

1. Set weight resistance to desired level.

2. Set position control for upper or lower ABs isolation.

3. Press chest against pad and push weight forward with the upper body, concentrating on crunching the ABs.

B. MUSCLES TRAINED

1. Upper ABs

2. Lower ABs

Cybex—Rotary Torso

A. INSTRUCTIONS

1. Adjust seat height so that upper pads are positioned across shoulders.

2. Place legs securely against the adductor pads, and select a comfortable foot position.

3. Release upper pull-button and move exercise arm to desired start position. The start position is adjustable in fifteen-inch increments.

4. Maintain contact with chest pad and grasp handles.

5. Lift weight by rotating torso slowly through the complete range of motion.

6. Pause briefly in the lifted position, then slowly lower the weight to the start position with a smooth, controlled motion.

7. Move pull-button to start position on opposite side, and repeat the exercise for other side of torso.

B. MUSCLES TRAINED

1. Internal obliques

2. External obliques

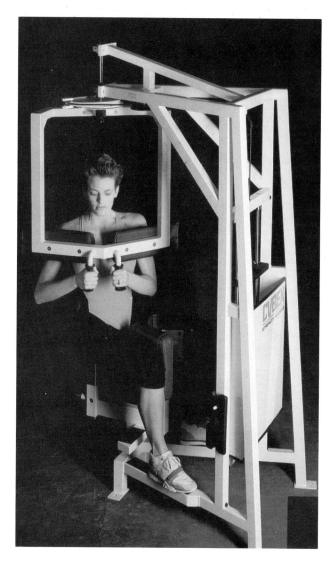

Cybex—Abdominal Machine

A. INSTRUCTIONS

1. Adjust seat height (align chest pad just below clavicle).
2. Select foot position. If front foot plate is chosen, adjust its height so that knee angle is 90 degrees.
3. Secure feet under instep straps or behind instep pads.
4. Place hands on top of thighs or on exercise bar.
5. Lift weight with smooth, controlled movements.
6. Pause briefly in the lifted position.
7. Slowly lower weight to start position.

B. MUSCLES TRAINED

1. Rectus abdominis

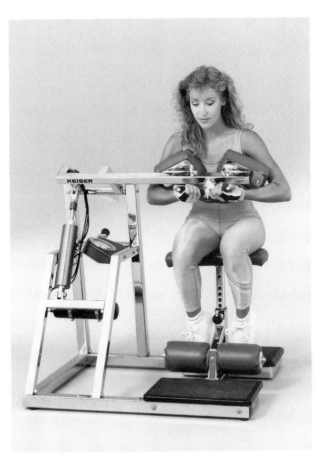

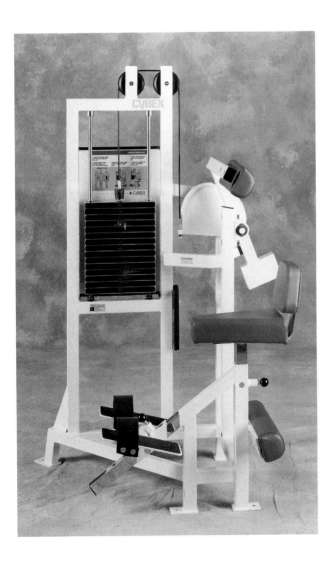

Keiser—Manual Abdominal

A. INSTRUCTIONS

1. Adjust the seat so the chest pads fit comfortably on the upper part of your chest.
2. Place your feet behind the leg-roller cushions.
3. Grasp the handgrips and select resistance with the thumb controls. The right thumb button increases resistance. The left button decreases resistance.
4. Lightly grasp the handgrips and bend forward, trying to bring your shoulders to your hips. Do not use your hip muscles during exercise. Move the exercise arm in a controlled manner through your full range of motion.

B. MUSCLES TRAINED

1. Rectus abdominis

LifeCircuit

A. INSTRUCTIONS

1. Adjust seat height so that the chest pads are positioned comfortably below the collarbone on the sternum.

2. Place body weight on seat pad, allowing the lower back to rest against the seat back.

3. Select program, press ENTER.

4. Grip handles, using a palms-up grip.

5. Keep feet firm to the floor.

6. Do not lean away from chest pads.

7. Begin exercise, moving lever arm at a smooth, controlled pace throughout the range of motion of the positive phase of the exercise. Do the same for the negative phase at a slightly slower rate.

B. MUSCLES TRAINED

1. Rectus abdominis

2. External obliques

3. Internal obliques

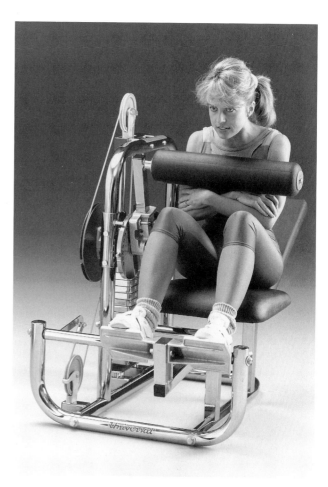

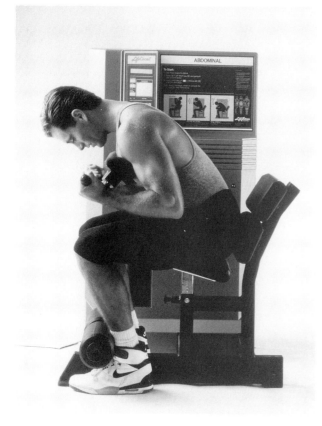

Universal—Abdominal Crunch

A. INSTRUCTIONS

1. Assume a semireclining position on machine with balls of feet on foot pedals.

2. Hips should be aligned with pivot point of the resistance arm.

3. Adjust resistance arm pad to a comfortable height and position against the chest.

4. Rest hands across the body below the pad, or over the pad toward shoulders.

5. Inhale and start moving the upper body (and the resistance arm pad) forward.

6. Continue bringing the upper body toward the knees (foot pedals will simultaneously bring knees toward upper body).

7. Exhale toward completion of the crunch.

8. Inhale while lowering weights under control to starting position.

B. MUSCLES TRAINED

1. Rectus abdominis

Nautilus—Lower Abdominal

A. INSTRUCTIONS

1. Sit in machine.

2. Make sure your hips are aligned with the axis of rotation of the movement arm. The area is marked with a red dot.

3. Fasten seat belt across thighs.

4. Lie back in reclining position.

5. Grasp handles lightly.

6. Keep torso and head on seat back.

7. Flex hips smoothly by drawing knees to chest.

8. Pause. Lower slowly to starting position, allowing the weight stack to barely touch. Repeat.

B. MUSCLES TRAINED

1. Iliopsoas

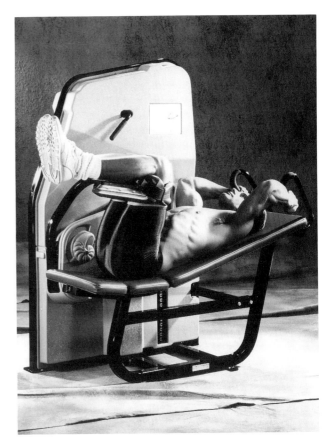

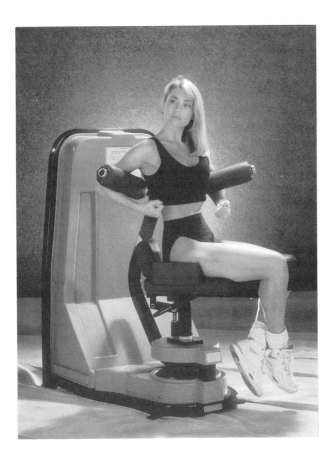

Nautilus—Rotary Torso

A. INSTRUCTIONS

1. Straddle the seat. Make sure the seat is adjusted and locked into the extreme right or left position. Use the handle on the right side to adjust the seat. Anchor your lower body by squeezing the pads between your knees.

2. Position your head and spinal column directly above the movement arm's pivot point.

3. Place your upper arms securely over the angled roller pads behind your back. Your elbows should be as close together as comfortably possible with your hands up.

4. Allow the back pressure of the movement arm to rotate you in one direction for a moderate stretch. Starting here, rotate to the opposite side.

5. Pause at completion, then return slowly to the starting position, and repeat.

6. After completing exercise, adjust the seat to the opposite side and lock in place. Repeat exercise for other side.

B. MUSCLES TRAINED

1. External obliques

2. Internal obliques

Nautilus—Abdominal (Next Generation)

A. INSTRUCTIONS

1. Adjust seat so navel aligns with red dot on side of machine.

2. Fasten seat belt across hips.

3. Place elbows on pads and grasp handles lightly.

4. Pull with elbows and shorten distance between ribs and pelvis. Do not try to pivot around hips.

5. Pause in contracted position. Keep shoulders against seat back.

6. Return slowly to starting position.

7. Repeat.

B. MUSCLES TRAINED

1. Rectus abdominis

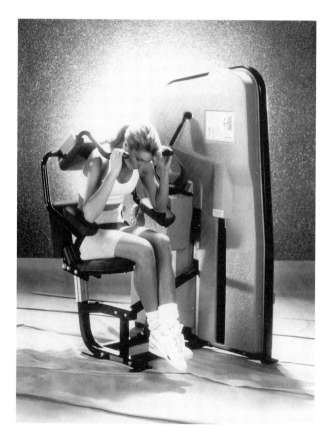

The New Home Machines

To some degree the craze has ended and cable television is no longer packed with infomercials for AB machines, but for almost two years you couldn't turn on your TV without seeing an advertisement for a product to trim and tone your midsection. Most of these products have been exposed for their false claims. The only machine that's shown staying power is the AB Roller.

TRAINING TIPS FOR AB ROLLERS:

What the following checklist boils down to is you are still responsible for the integrity of the movement. The machine doesn't magically solve all the problems and do all the work for you. It creates a new set of problems. The danger with the AB Roller is the possible misconception that all you have to do is get in it and rock and roll. The truth is you are still responsible for the exercise. And the fact that you are adjusting to a machine, which can't give you detailed feedback like your body, makes these potential problems more difficult. When using an AB Roller you need to focus even more on your basic technique, plus keep the following guidelines in mind:

1. Make sure the neck pad does not drive your head toward your chest, putting strain on your neck. This is the same effect as pulling your neck forward with your hands. Remember you need to keep a fist's distance between your chin and chest.

2. Don't push the Roller down with your elbows.

3. Don't push the Roller down with your hands or squeeze the Roller tightly with your hands.

4. Make sure the entire unit doesn't creep forward.

5. Let your neck relax into the pad, as if it were your hands.

6. You control the Roller; don't let the Roller control you. In other words, don't let momentum take over. You need to control both the upward and downward phases of the movement.

AB Trainer Basics

The following instructions and exercise guidelines describe the basic movements for using a Roller safely and effectively. So the next time you see a Roller at your gym don't feel intimidated, hop on and give it a try.

GETTING STARTED:

1. Lie flat on your back with your knees bent so your feet are flat on the floor. Rest your head comfortably on the headrest so the bottom of the headrest just touches the top of your shoulders.

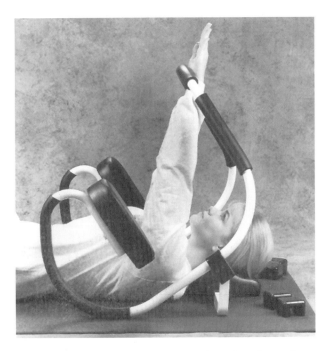

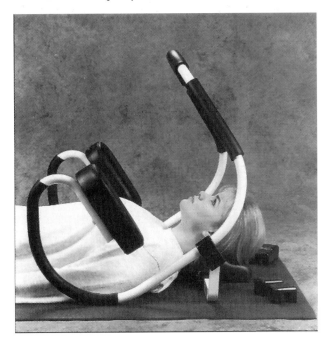

2. Extend arms through the center of the AB Trainer, placing arms against the center padded grip. Slowly curl forward, keeping head and neck relaxed against the headrest. Hold the curl at the top of the crunch, completely relax head and neck on the headrest, supporting the weight with abdominal muscles.

3. With head and neck completely relaxed, perform repetitions in slow controlled movement, beginning each repetition right before the headrest bar contacts the floor.

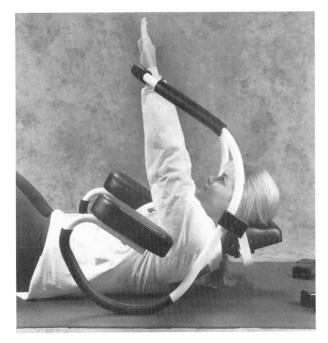

4. Do not lift head off headrest.

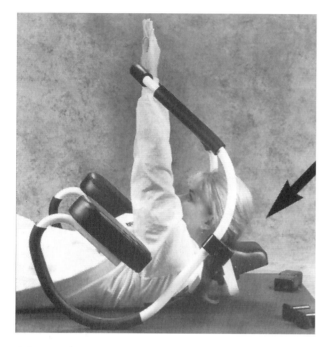

ARM POSITIONS:

Beginner: Arms extended through the center of the AB Trainer with arms against the center grip.

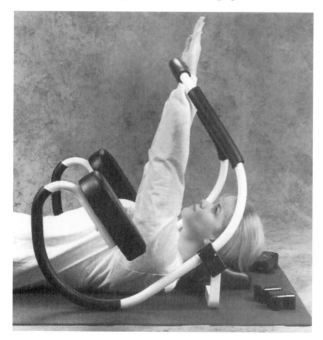

Advanced: Elbows on the elbow pads with hands against the outside (not grasping) of the handles.

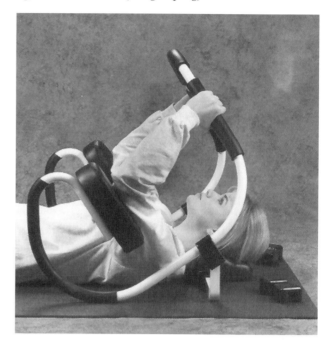

THE FOUR BASIC EXERCISES*

Basic Crunch: From starting position with either beginner or advanced hand position, slowly curl torso up with abdominal muscles, keeping head and neck relaxed on headrest throughout the entire range of motion. Pause momentarily at the end of the contraction and control return. Start next repetition right before the headrest bar touches the floor. Complete 10 to 15 repetitions (each rep should take 3 to 5 seconds). (See photos next page.)

---

* These tips and exercises come from Precise Fitness and the AB Trainer, one of the leading authorities on roller-training systems.

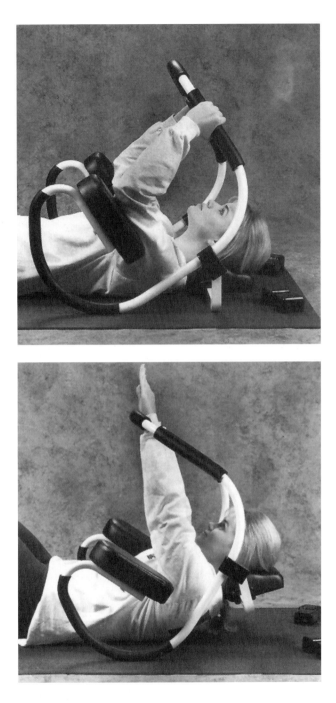

Reverse Crunch: Elevate legs from starting position (either bent or straight legs) with head and neck relaxed on the headrest and slightly raised off the floor. Pause momentarily at the top of the contraction, repeat. Do 10 to 15 repetitions (each rep should take 3 to 5 seconds).

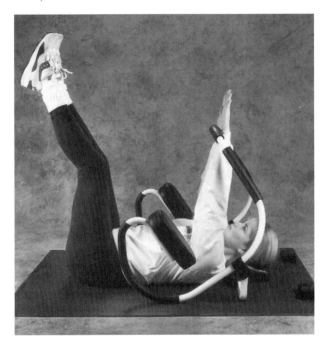

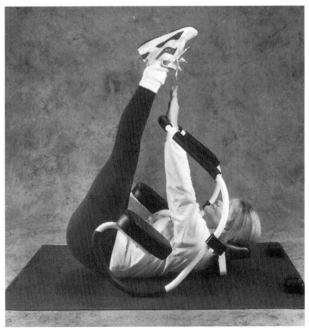

Side Crunch: From starting position, turn both legs to the right side. Cross the left arm over the right arm. Slowly curl torso up, remembering to relax the head and neck. Pause momentarily at the top of the contraction, repeat. Do 10 to 15 repetitions (each rep should take 3 to 5 seconds). Switch legs and hand positions and repeat.

Double Crunch: From the starting position, perform the basic and reverse crunch motions simultaneously. Pause momentarily at the top of the contraction, repeat. Do 10 to 15 repetitions (each rep should take 3 to 5 seconds).

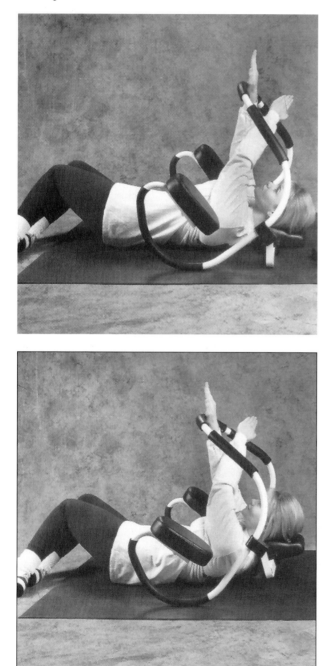

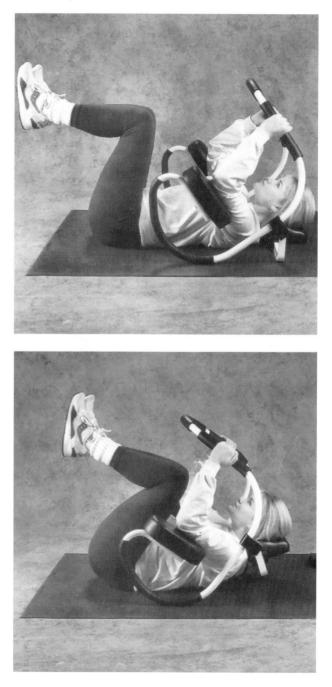

Videos

Another useful tool for working out in general, and AB exercises in particular, is workout videos. You can't always arrange to have a trainer or a friend on hand to help you work out, so videos can motivate and guide you when you're alone. Traditionally, only women have bought and used workout videos—probably because these videos were developed from daytime television exercise shows for housewives. Therefore men think that videos aren't macho enough and are embarrassed to use them—and, truth to tell, many videos do seem geared specifically for women. That's beginning to change, however. There are now dozens of workout videos on the market for every purpose and taste. There is no space here to review them all, but one video I can definitely recommend for any person serious about working out—either male or female—is *Abs of Steel*, produced by the Maier Group for their Men of Steel line. I have to admit this is not a completely unbiased recommendation—because I wrote and hosted the video! It contains some of the exercises and routines you'll find in this book, and I'm there in person to guide you through the exercises and give you trainer's tips. I think you'll find that *Abs of Steel* compliments this book quite nicely.

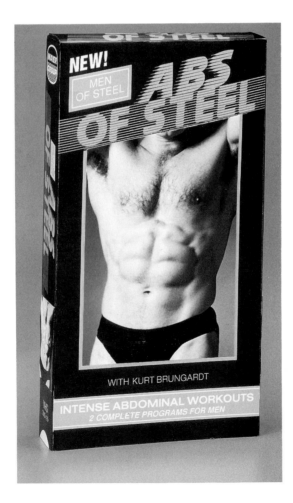

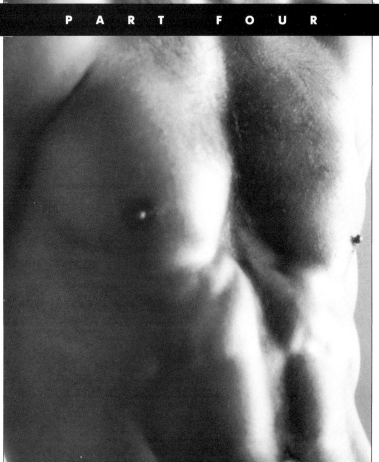

The Routines

ANATOMICALLY, ON THE HUMAN BODY, WHERE IS THE WAIST?

As an anatomical part, the waist doesn't exist. It was a term created
by the fashion industry for measurements.

CHAPTER SIXTEEN

Introduction to the Routines

This section offers a variety of routines to train your ABs for beauty, strength, and sports. The core of this section is Chapter 18: "The Complete Multi-Level System." This is one of the most extensive AB training programs ever developed. It guides you day by day, week by week, through a four-level program. But if you feel bogged down by such an extensive program, you can jump right into Chapter 17 and the "Get Started Now System." This progressive three-level program cuts right to the chase with challenging routines for all fitness levels.

In Chapter 19 you will find specialized routines for lower back sufferers and pregnancy, and proven workouts from the nation's leading fitness experts. You will also find routines to help you improve your favorite sports, such as golf, tennis, and skiing. And finally,

Chapter 20 will teach how to design a fitness program to fit your changing needs and goals.

Maintenance Routines

A maintenance routine allows you to maintain the benefits you have worked to achieve. If you finish a level and don't want to move on to the next, then you need a maintenance routine. For each level, you can maintain your results by following the routine of the last day of the level. For example, if you just wanted the health benefits of Level 1, you would follow the workout of Day 4, Week 6, three times a week. In most cases, it doesn't take as much work to maintain as it does to build. If you feel like increasing the intensity of your maintenance workouts while staying at the same level you can simply increase your workouts to five or six times a week. In ultimate ABs, you are already exercising six days a week.

As you become more advanced, maintenance becomes more complicated. If you complete Level 3 or 4, you need to look at Chapter 20, "Creating Your Own Routine," to define your next step. In any maintenance program, there will be deterioration over time. You cannot sustain the same fitness level for extended periods of time. Your body will eventually grow complacent to your maintenance routine. It's not a magic formula. What it *will* do is maintain the benefits you have worked to achieve.

Advancement

Everyone will progress at different speeds. The important thing is never to go on to the next level until you have achieved the goals of the previous level. The levels are designed in six-week increments. But if it takes you eight or ten weeks or longer to reach the goal of that level, then stay with it.

And don't forget, to achieve the look you want, you need to follow a healthy diet, cut down your fat content, and do cardiovascular work three to four times a week.

Substitutions

If there is an exercise in the system you can't do for whatever reason—back pain, lack of equipment, inability to correctly perform the exercise, etc.—then substitute. You need to choose an exercise that works the same area(s), has the same difficulty level, and isn't already in the routine. If you have exhausted all options, you can repeat an exercise that is already in the routine that fits this criteria.

Planning Your Workouts

Each level of both systems stands on its own and leads progressively into the next level. Depending on your needs and goals, you can stop at any level and go on a maintenance program, or push to the next level. Most of you will be able to start at Level 1. If this is too difficult then begin with the pre-conditioning phase.

During the pre-conditioning phase, you need to take a day off in between workouts. During Levels 1, 2, and 3, you need to take a day off between each two-day grouping. If you occasionally have to do your workouts back-to-back because of your schedule, this is okay. During ultimate ABs, if you miss a day, just pick it up the following day.

CHAPTER SEVENTEEN

Get Started Now System

Get Started: The Simple System

The following system is a simplified version of the more extensive system in Chapter 18. The repetitions prescribed for each level are goals. You may not be able to achieve them right away. The most important thing is to focus on strict technique. When you can easily complete the level's recommended reps, then move on to the next level.

BEGINNER ABS

EXERCISES	REPS	REST
1. Bent-Leg Hip Raises (page 90)	20	30 sec.
2. Reverse Sit-ups (page 179)	25	30 sec.
3. Side Jackknife: Modified (page 111)	20 each side	30 sec.
4. Crossovers (page 144)	20 each side	30 sec.
5. Crunches: Knees Bent (page 129)	25	30 sec.
6. Crunches: Frog Legs (page 134)	20	30 sec.

INTERMEDIATE ABS

EXERCISES	REPS	REST
1. Seated Knee Raises (page 94)	20	5 sec.
2. Hip Raises (page 88)	25	5 sec.
3. Bent-Leg Hip Raises (page 90)	25	5 sec.
4. Bicycles (page 101)	15 each side	5 sec.
5. Side Jackknife (page 112)	25 each side	5 sec.
6. Crossovers (page 144)	25 each side	5 sec.
7. Toe Touches (page 132)	10	5 sec.
8. Crunches: Knees Bent (page 129)	25	5 sec.
9. Crunches: Frog Legs (page 134)	25	5 sec.

EXERCISES	REPS	REST
3. Crunches: Knees Bent, on Incline Board (page 129)	25	5 sec.
4. Hanging Leg Raises (page 102)	25	5 sec.
5. Bicycles (page 101)	25 each side	5 sec.
6. Toe Touches: V Spread (page 161)	25	5 sec.
7. Hip Raises (page 88)	25	5 sec.
8. Oblique Crunches (page 159)	25 each side	5 sec.
9. Crunches: Knees Up (page 130)	25	5 sec.
10. Reverse Crunches (page 86)	25	5 sec.
11. Elbow to Hip (page 126)	25 each side	5 sec.
12. Crunches: Knees Up, Spread (page 138)	25	5 sec.

ADVANCED ABS: 15 MINUTES TO ULTIMATE ABS

EXERCISES	REPS	REST
1. Hanging Leg Raises with a Cross (page 184)	20	5 sec.
2. Side Jackknife (page 112)	25 each side	5 sec.

Note: Hold an isometric contraction for ten seconds at the end of each exercise.

The Complete Multi-Level System

Preconditioning Phase: The First Step

This level is designed for those who have never exercised before or who haven't exercised for a long time. It is a low-intensity, gradual program designed to build confidence and a strength base to prepare you for the rigors of Level 1. Just a few minutes, three times a week, will prepare you for that step. It is of primary importance to concentrate on proper technique. Relax and have fun. Don't get frustrated if the movements feel awkward at first. It just takes a while to get used to exercising again. You'll make progress in every workout.

Week 1
Days 1, 2, and 3

EXERCISES	SETS	REPS	REST
1. Modified Knee Raises (page 93)	1	1–5	30 sec.
2. Crossovers (page 144)	1	1–5	30 sec.
3. Crunches: Knees Up (page 130)	1	1–5	30 sec.

Do not proceed to next level until five repetitions can be completed on all exercises.

Week 2
Days 1, 2, and 3

EXERCISES	SETS	REPS	REST
1. Modified Knee Raises (page 93)	2	1–5	30 sec.
2. Crossovers (page 144)	2	1–5	30 sec.
3. Crunches: Knees Up (page 130)	2	1–5	30 sec.

Do not proceed to next level until five repetitions can be completed on all exercises for both sets.

Week 3
Days 1, 2, and 3

EXERCISES	SETS	REPS	REST
1. Modified Knee Raises (page 93)	1	5–8	30 sec.
2. Crossovers (page 144)	1	5–8	30 sec.
3. Crunches: Knees Up (page 130)	1	5–8	30 sec.
4. Isometric AB Pushdowns*	1		

* Lying on your back, knees bent, feet flat on ground, place hands on stomach. From this position, push back into floor, squeeze your AB muscles tight, holding for:

Day 1: 5 sec. and relax.
Day 2: 7 sec. and relax.
Day 3: 10 sec. and relax.

Week 4
Days 1, 2, and 3

EXERCISES	SETS	REPS	REST
1. Modified Knee Raises (page 93)	1	9–10	30 sec.
2. Crossovers (page 144)	1	9–10	30 sec.
3. Crunches: Knees Up (page 130)	1	9–10	30 sec.
4. Isometric AB Pushdowns*	1		

* Lying on your back, knees bent, feet flat on ground, place hands on stomach. From this position, push back into floor, squeeze your AB muscles tight, holding for: 10 sec. and relax.

Level 1: The Foundation

AB Chat The purpose of Level 1 is to build a foundation by developing a strong and muscularly balanced abdominal wall. To achieve this goal, you need to devote about five minutes a day, four times a week, to your ABs. A base of abdominal strength is necessary for good posture. Good posture will allow your whole body (internal organs, circulatory system, energy flow, etc.) to function at a higher level. It will also take pressure off the lower back, relieving back pain. Your ABs will also look and feel firmer.

Week 1
Days 1 and 2

EXERCISES	REPS	REST
1. Modified Knee Raises (page 93)	10	60 sec.
2. Crossovers (page 144)	10	60 sec.
3. Crunches: Knees Up (page 130)	10	60 sec.

Days 3 and 4

EXERCISES	REPS	REST
1. Same Exercises	12	60 sec.

Week 2
Days 1 and 2

EXERCISES	REPS	REST
1. Same Exercises	15	45 sec.

Days 3 and 4

EXERCISES	REPS	REST
1. Same Exercises	20	45 sec.

AB Chat The most important thing at this stage of your training is patience. It may not seem like you are doing much or seeing any results. Just stick with it, workout by workout—enjoy the process, love the struggle. The most important thing about exercising is consistency over time. Doing a little bit adds up. Be patient and stay with it! The results will come.

Now that you are feeling more confident, it is time to take your exercising to the next stage of awareness. The next two weeks concentrate on the finer points of exercise technique and feeling the muscles work: As you start to feel more confident in your technique, let the mind and the body come together.

Week 3
Days 1 and 2

EXERCISES	REPS	REST
1. Reverse Crunches (page 86)	10	45 sec.
2. Crossovers (page 144)	20	45 sec.
3. Crunches: Knees Up (page 130)	20	45 sec.

Days 3 and 4

EXERCISES	REPS	REST
1. Bent-Leg Hip Raises (page 90)	10	45 sec.
2. Reverse Crunches (page 86)	15	45 sec.
3. Crossovers (page 144)	20	45 sec.
4. Crunches: Knees Up (page 130)	20	45 sec.

AB Chat As you start your fourth week, you have probably experienced the feeling of not wanting to work out, of feeling weak, and of not reaching the recommended reps on all your exercises. There are days when you will experience setbacks. But setbacks aren't what they appear to be. A setback is often a preparation for a step or two forward. The body works in cycles, so don't be discouraged or quit because of a setback. Most are a hidden preparation for advancement. Setbacks are a small price you pay for getting to the next level.

Week 4
Days 1 and 2

EXERCISES	REPS	REST
1. Bent-Leg Hip Raises (page 90)	15	40 sec.
2. Reverse Crunches (page 86)	20	40 sec.
3. Crossovers (page 144)	25	40 sec.
4. Crunches: Knees Up (page 130)	25	40 sec.

Days 3 and 4

EXERCISES	REPS	REST
1. Bent-Leg Hip Raises (page 90)	20	40 sec.
2. Reverse Crunches (page 86)	25	40 sec.
3. Side Crunches (page 114)	10	40 sec.
4. Crossovers (page 144)	25	40 sec.
5. Crunches: Knees Up (page 130)	25	40 sec.

AB Chat As you approach the last two weeks of Level 1, it is important to have a little talk about *repetitions*. All repetition suggestions are just that . . . suggestions. When you have a breakdown in technique, you have done enough. That moment will be different from day to day. Here's why: How well did you sleep last night? What did you eat? What was your workout yesterday? Are you under a lot of stress at work or interpersonally? These are all important variables. It is unrealistic to demand robotic performance out of the human body. Disciplined? *Yes!* Specific? *Yes!* Challenging? *Yes!* Did I do my best? *Yes!*

Week 5
Days 1 and 2

EXERCISES	REPS	REST
1. Bent-Leg Hip Raises (page 90)	20	35 sec.
2. Reverse Crunches (page 86)	25	35 sec.
3. Side Crunches (page 114)	15	35 sec.
4. Crossovers (page 144)	25	35 sec.
5. Crunches: Knees Up (page 130)	25	35 sec.

Days 3 and 4

EXERCISES	REPS	REST
1. Bent-Leg Hip Raises (page 90)	20	30 sec.
2. Reverse Crunches (page 86)	25	30 sec.
3. Side Crunches (page 114)	20	30 sec.
4. Crossovers (page 144)	25	30 sec.
5. Crunches: Knees Up (page 130)	25	30 sec.

AB Chat As you push toward the finish of Level 1, if you're a smoker or a drinker, you may be wondering how this affects your workouts. Some of you may have recently quit smoking and put on weight. This may be the reason you bought this book. Regardless of how severe your habit is, starting to exercise is a positive first step toward controlling the habit.

This book is not about moral dogma. When it comes to bad habits, we all know better and worse. You know the negative health effects of smoking and drinking. The mission of this book is not to tell you to quit smoking or drinking. Changing is a matter of choice. No one can ultimately force you to do anything. It is nearly impossible to change your life all at once. It is a step-by-step process. As you start to exercise regularly and become more in tune with your body, certain physically harmful habits will begin to naturally fall by the wayside.

When controlling habits, think of just cutting back at first. Moderation is the best method. Don't beat yourself up over moments of weakness. Human frailty is not a sin. One good habit will naturally beget another good habit. Once you're on the right track, things will start to take care of themselves.

Week 6
Days 1 and 2

EXERCISES	REPS	REST
1. Bent-Leg Hip Raises (page 90)	20	30 sec.
2. Reverse Crunches (page 86)	25	30 sec.
3. Side Crunches (page 114)	20	30 sec.
4. Crossovers (page 144)	25	30 sec.
5. Crunches: Knees Up (page 130)	25	30 sec.
6. Crunches: Frog Legs (page 134)	10	30 sec.

Days 3 and 4

EXERCISES	REPS	REST
1. Bent-Leg Hip Raises (page 90)	20	30 sec.
2. Reverse Crunches (page 86)	25	30 sec.
3. Side Crunches (page 114)	25	30 sec.
4. Crossovers (page 144)	25	30 sec.
5. Crunches: Knees Up (page 130)	25	30 sec.
6. Crunches: Frog Legs (page 134)	20	30 sec.

Level 2: Bringing Out the Cuts

AB Chat The purpose of this level is to increase the endurance in your ABs and bring out more definition. You need to make about an eight-to-ten-minute commitment four times a week to achieve this goal. Your increased intensity will also help improve your general fitness level. You will burn more calories and improve your performance in sports and other recreational activities.

Week 1
Days 1 and 2

EXERCISES	REPS	REST
1. Hip Raises (page 88)	10	30 sec.
2. Bent-Leg Hip Raises (page 90)	25	30 sec.
3. Modified Side Jackknives (page 111)	10	30 sec.
4. Crossovers (page 144)	25	30 sec.
5. Crunches: Bent Knee (page 129)	25	30 sec.
6. Crunches: Frog Legs (page 134)	20	30 sec.

Days 3 and 4

EXERCISES	REPS	REST
1. Hip Raises (page 88)	15	30 sec.
2. Bent-Leg Hip Raises (page 90)	25	30 sec.
3. Modified Side Jackknives (page 111)	15	30 sec.
4. Crossovers (page 144)	25	30 sec.
5. Crunches: Bent Knee (page 129)	25	30 sec.
6. Crunches: Frog Legs (page 134)	20	30 sec.

AB Chat Visualization. Now that you are feeling more comfortable with exercising, it is time to start using your mental powers. Start to develop an ideal image or snapshot of how you want your ABs to look. See this picture before every workout.

Week 2
Days 1 and 2

EXERCISES	REPS	REST
1. Hip Raises (page 88)	20	25 sec.
2. Bent-Leg Hip Raises (page 90)	25	25 sec.
3. Modified Side Jackknives (page 111)	20	25 sec.
4. Crossovers (page 144)	25	25 sec.
5. Crunches: Bent Knee (page 129)	25	25 sec.
6. Crunches: Frog Legs (page 134)	25	25 sec.

Days 3 and 4

EXERCISES	REPS	REST
1. Hip Raises (page 88)	25	20 sec.
2. Bent-Leg Hip Raises (page 90)	25	20 sec.
3. Modified Side Jackknives (page 111)	25	20 sec.
4. Crossovers (page 144)	25	20 sec.
5. Crunches: Bent Knee (page 129)	25	20 sec.
6. Crunches: Frog Legs (page 134)	25	25 sec.

Days 3 and 4

EXERCISES	REPS	REST
1. Hip Raises (page 88)	25	20 sec.
2. Bent-Leg Hip Raises (page 90)	25	20 sec.
3. Modified Side Jackknives (page 111)	25	20 sec.
4. Crossovers (page 144)	25	20 sec.
5. Crunches: Bent Knee (page 129)	25	20 sec.
6. Crunches: Frog Legs (page 134)	25	20 sec.

AB Chat It is important to understand how leverage is involved in ABs work. Abdominals are your center, and gravity is your resistance. Every other part of the body is a lever. Unlike a weight machine, you are not able to simply lower the resistance as you approach fatigue. Your arms and legs are your resistance, so don't be afraid to adjust your position, bending your knees or changing the position of your arms to suit your individual needs. Slightly bending a knee can help take the work load off your back. You might put a towel under your neck to help prevent tension or a pillow under your tailbone. Keep open to creative options.

Week 3
Days 1 and 2

EXERCISES	REPS	REST
1. Hip Raises (page 88)	25	15 sec.
2. Bent-Leg Hip Raises (page 90)	25	15 sec.
3. Modified Side Jackknives (page 111)	25	15 sec.
4. Crossovers (page 144)	25	15 sec.

5. Crunches: Bent Knee (page 129)	25	15 sec.
6. Crunches: Frog Legs (page 134)	25	15 sec.

Days 3 and 4

EXERCISES	REPS	REST
1. Hip Raises (page 88)	25	10 sec.
2. Bent-Leg Hip Raises (page 90)	25	10 sec.
3. Modified Side Jackknives (page 111)	25	10 sec.
4. Crossovers (page 144)	25	10 sec.
5. Crunches: Bent Knee (page 129)	25	10 sec.
6. Crunches: Frog Legs (page 134)	25	10 sec.

AB Chat It is time to start adding cardiovascular work to your training regimen. At this point a little means a lot. If you can just do cardio work once a week for ten minutes, that's a good start. The important thing is to establish the habit. Chapter 7, "Complete Wellness," gives guidelines for setting up a cardio program.

Week 4
Days 1 and 2

EXERCISES	REPS	REST
1. Hip Raises (page 88)	25	5 sec.
2. Bent-Leg Hip Raises (page 90)	25	5 sec.
3. Modified Side Jackknives (page 111)	25	5 sec.
4. Crossovers (page 144)	25	5 sec.
5. Crunches: Bent Knee (page 129)	25	5 sec.
6. Crunches: Frog Legs (page 134)	25	5 sec.

Days 3 and 4

EXERCISES	REPS	REST
1. Seated Knee Raises (page 94)	10	5 sec.
2. Hip Raises (page 88)	25	5 sec.
3. Bent-Leg Hip Raises (page 90)	25	5 sec.
4. Modified Side Jackknives (page 111)	25	5 sec.
5. Crossovers (page 144)	25	5 sec.
6. Crunches: Bent Knee (page 129)	25	5 sec.
7. Crunches: Frog Legs (page 134)	25	5 sec.

AB Chat This week concentrate on technique. Think of your exercises as dance movements. Be proud of your technique: Don't rest at the bottom of your movements; hold total contractions for a count; keep the movements controlled; don't jerk or bounce.

Week 5
Days 1 and 2

EXERCISES	REPS	REST
1. Seated Knee Raises (page 94)	15	5 sec.
2. Hip Raises (page 88)	25	5 sec.
3. Bent-Leg Hip Raises (page 90)	25	5 sec.
4. Bicycles (page 101)	10	5 sec.
5. Modified Side Jackknives (page 111)	25	5 sec.
6. Crossovers (page 144)	25	5 sec.
7. Crunches: Bent Knee (page 129)	25	5 sec.
8. Crunches: Frog Legs (page 134)	25	5 sec.

Days 3 and 4

EXERCISES	REPS	REST
1. Seated Knee Raises (page 94)	20	5 sec.
2. Hip Raises (page 88)	25	5 sec.
3. Bent-Leg Hip Raises (page 90)	25	5 sec.
4. Bicycles (page 101)	15	5 sec.
5. Modified Side Jackknives (page 111)	25	5 sec.
6. Crossovers (page 144)	25	5 sec.
7. Toe Touches (page 132)	10	5 sec.
8. Crunches: Bent Knee (page 129)	25	5 sec.
9. Crunches: Frog Legs (page 134)	25	5 sec.

AB Chat This week focus on the mental side of training. Besides seeing your snapshot before every workout, concentrate on the mind-muscle link. Really put your mind in the muscle and feel the contraction in every repetition. Start to train your mind to be in the moment, committed to the task at hand, not going over all the errands you have to do after working out.

Week 6
Days 1 and 2

EXERCISES	REPS	REST
1. Seated Knee Raises (page 94)	20	No Rest
2. Hip Raises (page 88)	25	No Rest
3. Bent-Leg Hip Raises (page 90)	25	No Rest
4. Bicycles (page 101)	20	No Rest
5. Modified Side Jackknives (page 111)	25	No Rest

6. Crossovers (page 144)	25	No Rest
7. Toe Touches (page 132)	15	No Rest
8. Crunches: Bent Knee (page 129)	25	No Rest
9. Crunches: Frog Legs (page 134)	25	No Rest

Days 3 and 4

EXERCISES	REPS	REST
1. Seated Knee Raises (page 94)	20	No Rest
2. Hip Raises (page 88)	25	No Rest
3. Bent-Leg Hip Raises (page 90)	25	No Rest
4. Bicycles (page 101)	20	No Rest
5. Modified Side Jackknives (page 111)	25	No Rest
6. Crossovers (page 144)	25	No Rest
7. Toe Touches (page 132)	20	No Rest
8. Crunches: Bent Knee (page 129)	25	No Rest
9. Crunches: Frog Legs (page 134)	25	No Rest

Level 3: Washboard ABs

AB Chat The purpose of Level 3 is twofold: It incorporates both strength days and endurance days, building on the previous levels. You will need to commit about twenty minutes four times a week to achieve these goals. In this level, you are starting to sculpt your ABs. One of the changes in this level is increasing intensity by using more difficult exercises. You will see the size of your muscles increase slightly, bringing out the layered-washboard look. As you strive for the more chiseled look, diet and cardiovascular

work become more important. **Remember: Rest only between exercises, not between sets.**

Week 1
Days 1, 2, 3, and 4

EXERCISES	SETS	REPS	REST
1. Seated Leg Raises (page 190)	2	20	30
2. Oblique Crunches (page 159)	2	20	30
3. Cable Crunches (page 141)	2	20	30
4. Incline Reverse Crunches (page 86)	2	15	30
5. Incline Side Leg Raises (page 109)	2	15	30
6. Crunches: Legs Straight Out (page 133)	2	20	30

To conclude, hold a 10 sec. isometric contraction after the last exercise.

AB Chat If you are going to get the definition you want, you have to watch your diet. This week make it your goal to become more aware of what you eat. Read labels. Keep a food diary. See how foods affect your energy level. Then try to establish one new habit. Cut out some of the fat in your diet. Go from 2 percent milk to skim. Cut out desserts. Don't go back for seconds. Drink an extra glass of water. Read the diet chapter in this book!

Week 2
Days 1, 2, 3, and 4

EXERCISES	SETS/REPS	REST
1. Leg Raises (page 95)	2 × 25	30
2. Oblique Crunches (page 159)	2 × 25	30
3. Cable Crunches (page 144)	2 × 25	30

4. Incline Reverse Crunches (page 86)	2×25	30
5. Incline Side Leg Raises (page 109)	2×25	30
6. Crunches: Legs Straight Out (page 133)	2×25	30

To conclude, hold a 10 sec. isometric contraction after the last exercise.

> **AB Chat** Use your new powers of concentration to try the progressive relaxation techniques on pages 18–19. Try relaxing after each workout this week. After you have reached a relaxed state, visualize your ideal ABs. This technique is also great for relieving stress.

Week 3
Days 1 and 3

EXERCISES	REPS	REST
1. Hanging Knee Raises (page 99)	10	No Rest
2. Hanging Knee Raises with Cross (page 184)	10	No Rest
3. Side Jackknife (page 112)	20	No Rest
4. Bicycles (page 145)	20	No Rest
5. Incline Crunches (lowest) (page 129)	20	No Rest
6. Seated Knee Raises: Bent Knee (page 94)	20	No Rest
7. Knee-ups: Double-Leg Cross (page 168)	20	No Rest
8. Oblique Crunches (page 159)	20	No Rest
9. Toe Touches: V Spread (page 161)	20	No Rest
10. Sit-ups: Bent Knee (page 174)	20	No Rest

Days 2 and 4

EXERCISES	SETS/REPS
1. Seated Knee Raises (page 94)	3×15

2. Oblique Crunches (page 159)	3×20
3. Incline Crunches (page 129)	3×20
4. Hanging Leg Raises (page 102)	3×15
5. Side Jackknife (page 112)	3×20
6. Crunches: Raised Hip (page 135)	3×20

To conclude, hold a 10 sec. isometric contraction after the last exercise. Do entire routine. Rest 30 seconds. Repeat routine.

> **AB Chat** A long time ago, someone said, "No pain, no gain." AB work is different. Pain is a message. You need to listen closely to pain. Question the pain: "Where am I feeling it?" "How's my neck?" "How's my back?" "Is the pain spreading?" Push yourself, but be smart.

Week 4
Days 1 and 3

EXERCISES	REPS	REST
1. Hanging Leg Raises (page 102)	15	No Rest
2. Hanging Leg Raises with Cross (page 184)	15	No Rest
3. Side Jackknife (page 112)	25	No Rest
4. Bicycles (page 145)	25	No Rest
5. Incline Crunches (page 129)	25	No Rest
6. Seated Knee Raises (page 94)	25	No Rest
7. Knee-ups: Double-Leg Cross (page 168)	25	No Rest
8. Oblique Crunches (page 159)	25	No Rest
9. Toe Touches: V Spread (page 161)	25	No Rest
10. Sit-ups: Bent Knee (page 174)	25	No Rest

Week 4
Days 2 and 4

EXERCISES	SETS/REPS
1. Seated Knee Raises (page 94)	3×20
2. Oblique Crunches (page 159)	3×25
3. Incline Crunches (page 129)	3×25
4. Hanging Leg Raises (page 102)	3×20
5. Side Jackknife (page 112)	3×25
6. Crunches: Raised Hip (page 135)	3×25

Do entire routine. Rest 30 seconds. Repeat routine.

> **AB Chat** Make it a goal this week to do cardio-vascular work three times. This is an important habit to establish. Not only for your ABs, but for your overall health and longevity. Again, work with the cardio program outlined in Chapter 8.

Week 5
Days 1 and 3:

Perform all seven exercises without rest, then rest one minute and perform again.

EXERCISES	REPS	REST
1. Side Jackknife (page 112)	20	No Rest
2. Hanging Half Leg Raises (page 102)	5–8	No Rest
3. Corkscrews (page 147)	20	No Rest
4. Incline Side Jackknife (page 112)	10	No Rest
5. Crunches: Raised Hip with Twist (page 157)	20	No Rest
6. Crunches: Raised Hip (page 157)	20	No Rest
7. Bicycles (page 145)	60	

To conclude, hold a 10 sec. isometric contraction after the last exercise.

Days 2 and 4:

Use a weight that will still allow you to isolate muscle, but also brings you to momentary muscular exhaustion for the prescribed number of repetitions. Rest 30 seconds between sets and between exercises.

EXERCISES	SETS/REPS	REST
1. Seated Knee Raises (page 94)	2×12	30 sec.
2. Hanging Leg Raises (page 102)	2×10	30 sec.
3. Russian Twists (page 162)	2×10	30 sec.
4. Toe Touches: V Spread (page 161)	2×10	30 sec.
5. Incline Crunches (page 129)	2×12	30 sec.
6. Sit-ups: Feet Up (page 176)	2×10	30 sec.

> **AB Chat** Although we are taught from birth to avoid it, failure is not a dirty word. In fact, fitness is dedicated to failure. It is the failure of a muscle to complete a task that dictates the level of strength gained. How can you get stronger if you don't test limits? You have to learn to love the struggle. In a way, failure is always victory in defeat. It is always better than stopping short.

Week 6
Days 1 and 3:

Perform all seven exercises in a continuous manner, then rest thirty seconds and perform again.

EXERCISES	REPS	REST
1. Side Jackknife (page 112)	30	No Rest
2. Hanging Half Leg Raises (page 102)	10–15	No Rest
3. Corkscrews (page 147)	30	No Rest

4. Incline Double-Leg Jackknife (page 113)	15	No Rest
5. Crunches: Raised Hip (page 135)	30	No Rest
6. Bicycles (page 145)	80	

Days 2 and 4:

Use a weight that will still allow you to isolate muscle, but also brings you to momentary muscular exhaustion for the prescribed number of repetitions. Rest 30 seconds between sets and exercises. Try to increase the weight from the previous week.

EXERCISES	SETS/REPS	REST
1. Seated Knee Raises (page 94)	2 × 12	30 sec.
2. Hanging Leg Raises (page 102)	2 × 10	30 sec.
3. Russian Twists (page 162)	2 × 10	30 sec.
4. Toe Touches: V Spread (page 161)	2 × 10	30 sec.
5. Incline Crunches (page 129)	2 × 12	30 sec.
6. Sit-ups: Feet Up (page 176)	2 × 10	30 sec.

Note: Hold 10-second isometric contraction on the last rep of each exercise.

Level 4: Ultimate ABs

AB Chat The purpose of this level is to train the ABs in a very specific and refined way. Each workout targets a specific area of the ABs. Your training schedule is now six times a week. Each area is also broken up with an endurance day and a strength day (using light weights). The goal is to bring your ABs into peak condition.

INSTRUCTIONS:
Weeks 1–3: Days 1, 2, and 3 are performed with no rest between exercises. On Week 3, rest for two minutes and repeat the entire circuit with no rest between exercises.

Weeks 1–3: Days 4, 5, and 6 are performed as follows:

Week 1: Two sets of each exercise with thirty seconds' rest between sets.

Week 2: Same as Week 1.

Week 3: Three sets of each exercise with thirty seconds' rest between sets.

AB Chat If you need more rest in the beginning, that's fine. But set your goal for the prescribed thirty seconds.

On any weight day, if you can't use a weight or if you're not strong enough (remember to use very light weight when training your ABs), then substitute five-second isometric holds on every fifth repetition. It's important to remember that using weights will have a tendency to add mass to your ABs. The same goes for Weeks 4, 5, and 6.

As you make your way through these last three weeks, it is important to really listen to your body. Your body goes through natural cycles of growth and rest. Your body thrives on both structure and change. Everybody's cycles are different. Ultimately, the goal is to train with your instincts and intuition. Your body will talk to you. It will tell you when to take an extra day off, when to go slow instead of risking an injury, and when to push through that extra repetition. It is your responsibility to know your body and be in touch with it. The more you work out, the more you take the time to stop and listen to it, the better you will get to know yourself.

INSTRUCTIONS:
Weeks 4–6 Days 1, 2, and 3:

Week 4: Every exercise without rest in between. Rest two minutes and repeat the circuit.

Week 5: Same as Week 4, except one minute thirty seconds between repeating the circuit.

Week 6: Same as above, except a minute's rest between repeating the sequence.

Days 4, 5, and 6:

Week 4: Two sets of each exercise with thirty seconds' rest between sets.

Week 5: Three sets with twenty seconds' rest between sets.

Week 6: Four sets with twenty seconds' rest between sets.

AB Chat After you have completed Ultimate ABs, it is important that you continually change your routine to keep it fresh and to achieve complete development.

WEEKS: 1, 2, AND 3
Lower ABs
Day 1: Endurance
Day 4: Weight

	ENDURANCE DAYS REPS DAY 1			STRENGTH (WEIGHT) DAYS REPS DAY 4		
EXERCISE	WEEK 1	WEEK 2	WEEK 3	WEEK 1	WEEK 2	WEEK 3
1. Hanging Leg Raises (page 102)	10	12	15	5	7	9
2. Hanging Leg Raises with Cross (page 106)	8	10	12	4	6	8
3. Incline Leg Raises (highest incline) (page 95)	20	25	30	10	12	15
4. Incline Knee Raises (highest incline) (page 91)	20	25	30	10	12	15
5. Seated Knee Raises (page 94)	20	25	30	10	12	15
6. Hip-ups (page 125)	20	25	30	10	12	15

Obliques
Day 2: Endurance
Day 5: Weight

	REPS DAY 2			REPS DAY 5		
EXERCISE	WEEK 1	WEEK 2	WEEK 3	WEEK 1	WEEK 2	WEEK 3
1. Side Jackknives (page 112)	12	15	20	5	8	12
2. Side Knee-ups (page 173)	15	20	25	8	10	12
3. Side Sit-ups: Roman Chair (page 115)	20	25	30	10	12	15
4. Oblique Crunches (page 159)	20	25	30	10	12	15
5. Crunches with a Twist (page 157)	20	25	30	10	12	15
6. Crunches with a Twist: Raised Hip (page 157)	25	30	35	10	12	15

Upper ABs
Day 3: Endurance
Day 6: Weight

	REPS DAY 3			REPS DAY 6		
EXERCISE	WEEK 1	WEEK 2	WEEK 3	WEEK 1	WEEK 2	WEEK 3
1. Incline Crunches (page 129)	15	20	25	10	12	15
2. Sit-ups: Feet Up (page 176)	15	20	25	10	12	15
3. Crunches: Raised Hip (page 135)	20	25	30	10	12	15
4. Toe Touches (page 132)	20	25	30	10	12	15
5. Crunches: Leg Straight Up, Spread (page 142)	20	25	30	10	12	15
6. Crunches: Knees Up (page 130)	20	25	30	10	12	15

WEEKS: 4, 5, AND 6
Day 1: Endurance
Day 4: Weight

	ENDURANCE DAYS			STRENGTH (WEIGHT) DAYS		
	REPS DAY 1			REPS DAY 4		
EXERCISE	WEEK 1	WEEK 2	WEEK 3	WEEK 1	WEEK 2	WEEK 3
1. Hanging Leg Raises (page 102)	15	17	20	9	10	12
2. Hanging Half Leg Raises (page 185)	10	15	20	8	10	12
3. Incline Corkscrews (page 147)	20	25	30	9	12	15
4. Leg Overs: Double Leg (page 124)	15	20	30	10	10	10
5. Knee-ups (page 167)	15	20	30	10	10	10
6. Seated Knee Raises (page 94)	20	25	30	10	10	10

Day 2: Endurance
Day 5: Weight

	REPS DAY 2			REPS DAY 5		
EXERCISE	WEEK 1	WEEK 2	WEEK 3	WEEK 1	WEEK 2	WEEK 3
1. Side Jackknives: on Incline (page 113)	10	15	20	6	9	12
2. Side Leg Raises: on Incline (page 109)	15	20	25	10	10	10
3. Side Sit-ups: Roman Chair (page 115)	10	15	20	10	10	10
4. Russian Twists (page 162)	30	40	50	15	15	15
5. Toe Touches: V Spread (page 161)	20	25	30	10	10	10
6. Inclined Crossovers (page 144)	25	30	35	10	10	10

Day 3: Endurance
Day 6: Weight

	REPS DAY 3			REPS DAY 6		
EXERCISE	WEEK 1	WEEK 2	WEEK 3	WEEK 1	WEEK 2	WEEK 3
1. Crunches: Knees Bent, Spread (page 137)	20	25	30	6	9	12
2. Toe Touches (page 132)	20	25	30	10	10	10
3. Incline Sit-ups (page 174)	15	20	25	10	10	10
4. Incline Crunches (page 129)	20	25	30	10	10	10
5. Crunches: Frog Legs (page 134)	20	25	30	10	10	10
6. Toe Touches: V Spread (page 161)	30	40	50	15	15	15

Workouts of the Pros and Specialized Routines

This chapter gives the AB routines of top fitness experts, bodybuilders, and professional strength coaches in their area of expertise. These specialized routines are geared toward specific groups and specific sports.

The Office Routine by Mike Brungardt and Kurt Brungardt

Mike Brungardt is on the board of directors of Strength Advantage, Inc. As a member of Strength Advantage, he has performed seminars at top health clubs and given clinics for fitness educators in schools throughout the country.

INTRODUCTION This routine is designed to give you an AB workout without ever leaving your office chair. You can do it during a break, right before lunch, or at the end of the day. It's also a fun way to work off a little stress.

PRE-CONDITIONING (2 WEEKS)

1. Single Knee Raises: Raise knee toward your chest
Week 1: 10 reps each leg
Week 2: 20 reps each leg

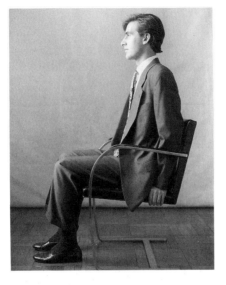 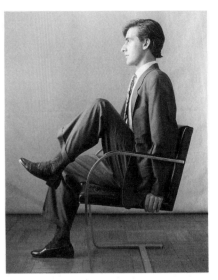

2. Elbow to Hip (Hold contraction for one count): Lower your elbow and rib cage toward your hip
Week 1: 10 reps each side
Week 2: 20 reps each side

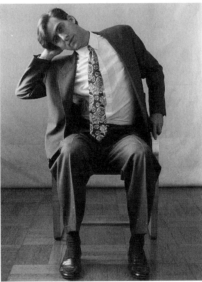

3. Seated Crunchdown: Crunch your rib cage toward your pelvis.
Week 1: 10 reps
Week 2: 20 reps

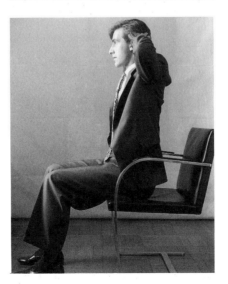 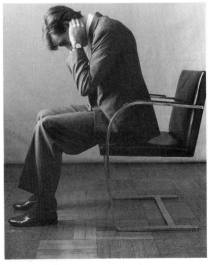

LEVEL 1 (3 WEEKS)

1. Knee Raises: Raise both knees toward your chest
Week 1: 10 reps
Week 2: 15 reps
Week 3: 20 reps

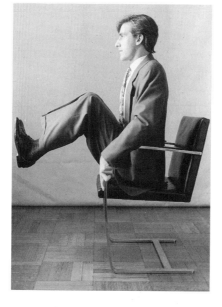
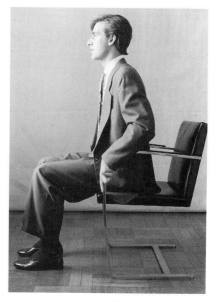

2. Crosses: Cross your opposite shoulder and knee toward each other.
Week 1: 10 reps each leg
Week 2: 15 reps each leg
Week 3: 20 reps each leg

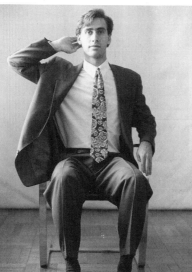
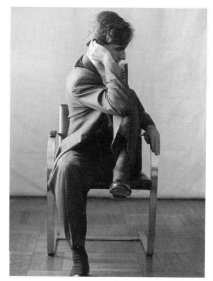

3. Elbow to Hip
Week 1 through 3: 20 reps each side

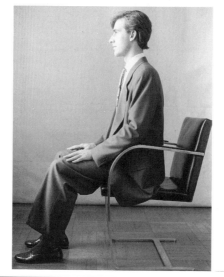
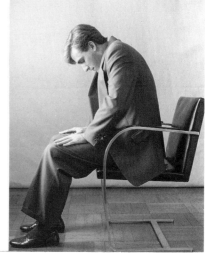

4. Iso Pushdowns (page 193)
   Week 1: 10 seconds
   Week 2: 10 seconds
   Week 3: 10 seconds

5. Quick Crunchdowns: From a seated position, hands behind your ears, crunch your rib cage down toward your pelvis. Same as Seated Crunchdown, but at a faster pace.
   Week 1: 10 reps
   Week 2: 15 reps
   Week 3: 20 reps

LEVEL 2

1. Leg Raises: From starting position in picture, raise your legs as high as you can while maintaining good form.
   Week 1: 10 reps
   Week 2: 15 reps
   Week 3: 20 reps

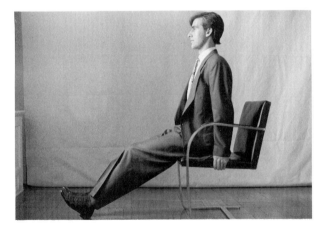 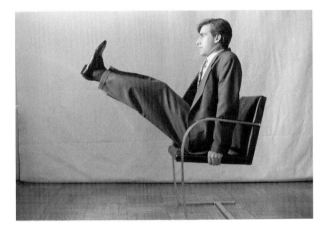

2. Knee Ups: Lean your torso back and then bring your knees and chest together.
   Week 1: 10 reps
   Week 2: 15 reps
   Week 3: 20 reps

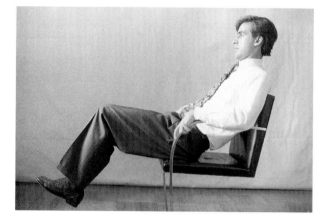 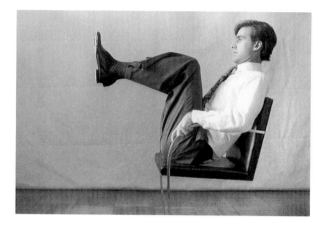

3. Incline Bicycles: Leaning back, bring your opposite elbows and knees together.
   Week 1: 10 reps
   Week 2: 15 reps
   Week 3: 20 reps

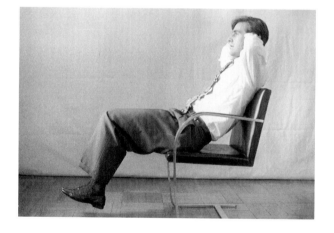 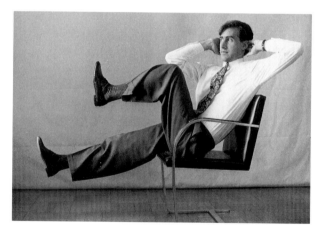

4. Elbow to Hip (page 126)
   Week 1: 20 reps each side
   Week 2: 20 reps each side
   Week 3: 20 reps each side

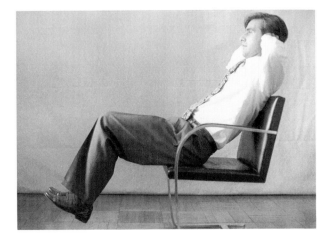
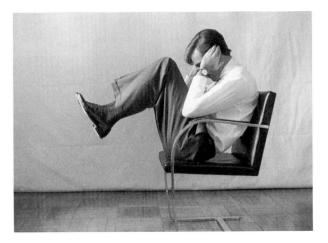

5. Elbow to Knee: Simultaneously bring your knees
and elbows together.
Week 1: 10 reps
Week 2: 15 reps
Week 3: 20 reps

LEVEL 3

1. Incline Leg Raises: Lean your torso back and
raise your legs as high as you can.
Week 1: 10 reps each leg
Week 2: 15 reps each leg
Week 3: 20 reps each leg

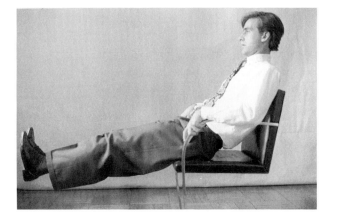
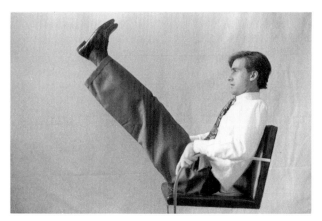

2. Knee-ups (page 167)
Week 1: 10 reps each leg
Week 2: 15 reps each leg
Week 3: 20 reps each leg

3. Double-Knee Crosses: Simultaneously, raising both knees, bring your opposite knee and shoulder toward each other.
Week 1: 10 reps each leg
Week 2: 15 reps each leg
Week 3: 20 reps each leg

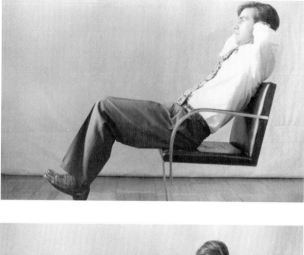

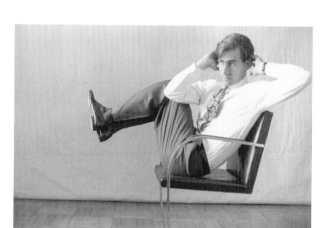

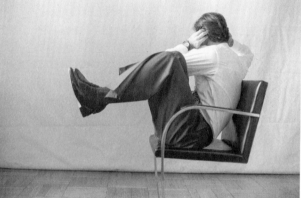

4. Incline Straight-Leg Crosses: Straighten one leg and then raise it toward your opposite shoulder as you bring your shoulder toward the knee.
Week 1: 10 reps each leg
Week 2: 15 reps each leg
Week 3: 20 reps each leg

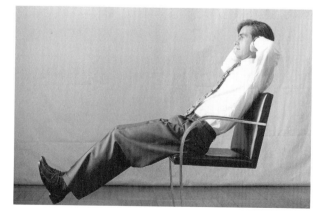

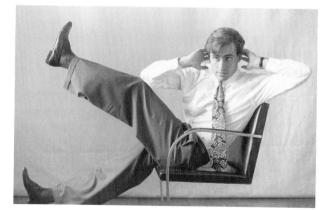

5. V-ups: Lean your torso back, then jacknife your torso and your legs toward each other, making a tight V.
Week 1: 10 reps
Week 2: 15 reps
Week 3: 20 reps

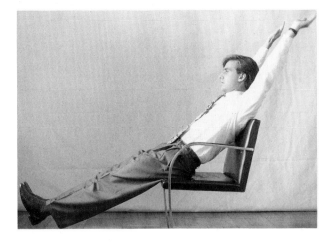 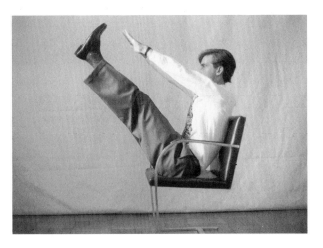

6. Elbow to Hip
Week 1: 20 reps on each side
Week 2: 20 reps on each side
Week 3: 20 reps on each side with a 10-second isometric hold on the last rep of the set.

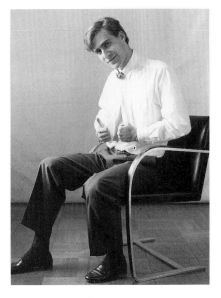

When you have completed Level 3, move up to thirty reps for each of the six exercises and finish with the ten-second Iso Pushdown. Then try to do this routine (thirty reps per exercise) three to four times a week.

Make sure you follow sound training technique: holding total contractions at the top of movement for a count of two, not resting at the bottom of movement, and focusing your mind on your ABs.

The Jeff Martin ABs Routine
by Jeff Martin

Jeff Martin is known worldwide to both students and instructors for his enthusiasm and innovative teaching methods, and as a fitness-industry leader.

THE ROUTINE If you follow this routine, not only will you have a flat, toned stomach with sculpted contours of definition, you will also build yourself a natural girdle of muscle so that you have no trouble holding your stomach in. The only way to work the oblique muscles is to perform twisting motions as in the Serratus Crunch. The Serratus Crunch works both the upper abdominal area and the intacostals.

THE EXERCISE POSITIONING Lie flat on your back on the floor or a mat. Wrap your legs around a flat exercise bench, Place your right leg over the bench and your left leg under the bench. Cross your legs at the ankles.

MOVEMENT Raise yourself up on your right side by lifting your shoulders and torso until you feel an intense contraction in your waist. Return to starting position and repeat the movement without resting until you have completed your set. Reverse the position of your legs and repeat the exercise for your left side. Repeat the exercises until you have done three sets for each side of your body.

ABS WISDOM
- Keep your mind focused on your sides—oblique abdominal muscles.
- Forcefully exhale as you lift up.
- Resist the temptation to jolt yourself off the floor in an effort to gain momentum and make the work easier. Be consistent and concentrate. Keep your abdominal muscles flexed throughout the movement.

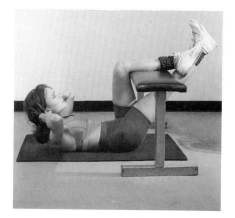

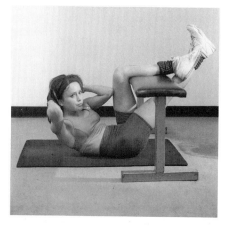

The Plus One ABs Routine
by Mike Motta

Michael Motta is the president and cofounder of Plus One Fitness Clinics, New York, New York. As a personal trainer for nine years in Manhattan, Mike has worked with Cher, Glenn Close, Bernadette Peters, Tom Cruise, Madonna, Calvin Klein, James Taylor, Robin Williams, and Joel Grey. Mike has a master's degree in exercise physiology, is certified by the American College of Sports Medicine, and is an adjunct faculty member of New York University's School of Continuing Education.

Plus One is a medically based health and fitness company that combines exercise science and sports medicine. In addition to employing an extensive staff of physical therapists, massage therapists, and exercise specialists, Plus One manages fitness centers for the Waldorf-Astoria Hotel, The New York Hilton Hotel, and Morgan Stanley & Company, Inc.

INTRODUCTION This is an intermediate/advanced routine for any trainee who wants some variety in his/her ABs exercises and a little challenge. The routine also incorporates exercises for the external obliques, the erector spinae, the lumbodorsal fascia, and the medial aspect of the latissimus dorsi. In combination, this group is often neglected and is essential for muscular balance (between back and abdominals) and good posture.

THE EXERCISES
1. The Rope Climb
- Lie flat on your back, knees bent, feet flat.
- Visualize a rope hanging from the ceiling and almost touching your chin.
- Reach up with arms extended, climb the imaginary rope with a hand-over-hand movement.
- Climb straight up, lifting only your head, neck, shoulders, and upper back off the floor only while contracting your abdominals.
- Climb for five seconds, then roll back down to the starting position.

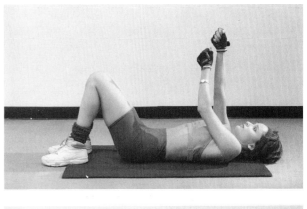

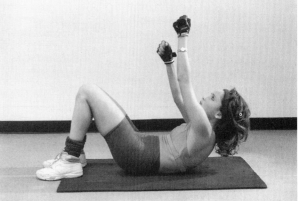

2. The "Over the Shoulder"

- Lie on your stomach with your head down, legs straight and looking to your left.
- Place your right hand behind your back with the palm up and the left arm at your side.
- While keeping your legs relaxed, lift your head, neck, chest. and upper stomach off the mat.
- As you lift, rotate slightly to the right, turn your head around (so you are looking over your right shoulder) and drive the right shoulder up and around. (NOTE: This exercise requires only a small amount of movement.)
- Concentrate on all the posterior muscles of the lower back and your external obliques in the right side as you lift.
- Then return to starting position in a slow and controlled fashion.
- Reverse direction above to perform reps for left side.

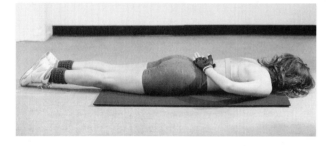

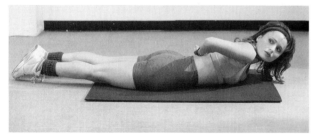

THE ROUTINE

Note: The second count refers to the duration of each rep, meaning your hand-over-hand movements. After sufficient warm-up and stretching:

1. Rope Climb

- 5 reps × 5 seconds (with 5 seconds' rest between reps)
- Rest 30 seconds.
- 7 reps × 7 seconds (with 7 seconds' rest between reps)

2. "Over the Shoulder"

- 5 reps to right
- 5 reps to left
- Rest 10 seconds.
- 10 reps to right
- 10 reps to left
- Roll over and pull both knees to chest for 10 seconds.

3. Rope Climb

- 10 reps for 6 seconds (with 6 seconds' rest between reps)
- Rest 30 seconds.
- 10 reps for 7 seconds (with 5 seconds' rest between reps)
- Rest 30 seconds.
- 5 reps for 10 seconds (with 5 seconds' rest between reps)

4. "Over the Shoulder"

- Same as above

ABS WISDOM The torso acts as your column of support between your lower body (the foundation) and your upper body (the roof). Adequate and balanced strength between all of the muscles of the torso is essential for this group to perform its functions as your pillar of support. You should concentrate on the function and stability of your torso in all your exercises. Use your torso strength to stabilize your hips while performing lower-body exercises and to stabilize your rib cage while performing upper-body exercises.

The Husky Circuit Routine by Rick Huegli

Rick Huegli is the University of Washington's head strength coach. He has responsibility for teaching, administering, and supervising the Husky strength program for all twenty-one intercollegiate sports. He supervised and planned the opening of Washington's expansive, state-of-the-art weight room in 1988. The facility ranks second among major colleges, with 10,700 square feet available. Up to three hundred athletes per day use the weight room at peak periods. This year, Huegli was honored as the National Strength and Conditioning Coach of the Year by his colleagues.

ABDOMINAL CIRCUIT ROUTINE The circuit consists of four exercises employing three to five circuits. The exercises are Knee-ups, Crunches, Russian Twists, and an exercise I call "Touch and Overhead." This circuit will involve emphases on the lower, upper, and oblique abdominals providing core strength. The routine is employed one to two times a week, providing from 330 to 550 abdominal efforts.

THE EXERCISES

1. Knee-ups (page 167)
Starting Position: Using a Roman chair apparatus, the athlete supports himself or herself on the forearms with the hands on the grips and the rest of the body in a vertical position.
The Movement: Lift the bent knees to a position where the thighs are parallel to the ground or as close to the chest as possible. Hold the position for a two count, then return to the starting position.

An advanced variation would be to keep the legs straight and raise them to a 90-degree angle in relation to the upper body forming an L position. Complete twenty to fifty reps per set.

ABS WISDOM Concentrate on contracting the lower abdominal muscles. Raise the legs with control, hold for a two count, and lower with control.

Upon completion of a set of Knee-ups, go immediately to the Crunches.

2. Crunches (page 129)
Starting Position: The Crunch can be done from a number of starting positions.
1. Begin by lying down with the knees bent, feet flat on the ground, the hands behind the head and the lower back always in contact with the ground.
2. Same as step 1, but with the feet and lower legs elevated in a parallel-to-the-ground position.
3. Same as step 1, but with the lower legs resting across a bench.
The Movement: Raise the shoulders and upper back about 30 degrees off the ground, bringing the chin to the chest and hold for a two count; then slowly return to the starting position. Complete fifty reps per set.

ABS WISDOM Do not pull with the arms against the back of the head. Concentrate on a two-count contraction initiated from the lower to the upper abdominals.

Upon completion of a set of Crunches, immediately go to the Russian Twist.

3. Russian Twists (page 162)
Starting Position: Begin by positioning the body in an inclined seated position with the feet flat on the floor secured by a partner or tucked under a piece of equipment for stability. Hold a medicine ball or other weight away from the body.
The Movement: Begin with a 10 kg medicine ball or a 5–10 lb. weight. Rotate the torso from side to side keeping the arms extended. Rotating from one side to the other constitutes one rep. Complete twenty reps per set.

ABS WISDOM Follow the path of the ball with the head and eyes and keep the butt in complete contact with the seated surface. Focus on rotating the torso with the oblique muscles rather than the shoulders.

Upon completion of a set of the Russian Twist, go immediately to the "Touch and Overhead" exercise.

4. "Touch and Overhead"

Starting Position: Begin by positioning the body in a shoulder-width squat stance holding a medicine hall with both hands.

The Exercise: With the ball held in front of the body, squat down, touching the ball to the floor between and just in front of the toes. In one accelerating movement, raise the ball simultaneously with the hips and shoulders. Explosively extend vertically through the hips, pulling the ball to the left overhead position, arms extended. Return to the floor position to repeat the move-

ment and extend to the right overhead position with the ball to complete two repetitions.

ABS WISDOM
- Maintain proper squat mechanics at the floor position (low back tight, neutral head position, shoulder-width foot stance, hips and shoulders move as a unit).
- Avoid overextending the back when pulling the ball through to the overhead position.
- Maintain extended-arm position throughout range of motion.

As with any circuit, you can vary repetitions, number of circuits, and the amount of time between exercises or circuits. I advise doing a complete circuit with a recovery period only as long as it takes to go from one exercise station to the next. Focus on proper technique and exercise tempo, and you will find this routine one that is quick and intense and hits the entire abdominal area.

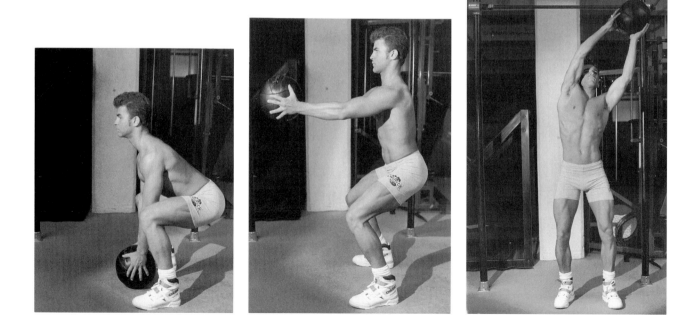

The Prenatal Routine
by Robin Mandel-Naylon

Robin Mandel-Naylon has her prenatal certificate from A.F.A.A. and she is also a member of I.D.E.A. She is owner of Quoque Fitness and program director of Crunch Fitness. She has her B.S. from SUNY Buffalo.

INTRODUCTION How can you maintain or develop strong ABs during pregnancy? First, check with your ob/gyn to make sure you are in good condition before starting any exercise program. You may begin this program during any part of your term. Working your ABs on your back (supine), however, is not recommended after the fifth or sixth month of your term.

It is important to work at your own level. This is not a time to push yourself to your limit. Do what feels comfortable.

THE TRIMESTERS I have set up an ABs program for your three different trimesters. The comfort of these positions may vary throughout your pregnancy, and because everyone is different, it is not essential to follow this program verbatim.

It is recommended during your first trimester to slightly decrease your exercise levels. I call this the settling and readjusting period. Because of nausea and morning sickness, it is better to take it a bit easy and resume increased levels during the second trimester.

Naturally, during your third trimester you will ease off and stay with isometrics or nothing at all. Again, everyone will vary, and you can stay with any section for as long as you feel comfortable.

THE EXERCISES

First and Second Trimester

1. Crunches with Single Leg

Lie on your back, right leg bent, foot flat on the ground, and left leg extended straight (knee unlocked). From this position, simultaneously raise your left leg and shoulders toward each other as you exhale. Hold the contraction at the top for a count, then release the leg and shoulder. Try not to touch the ground with your leg or head.

Recommendations: Begin with three sets of eight and work up to sixteen. Then try to do three more sets performing a constant pulse: starting with eight and working up to sixteen pulses.

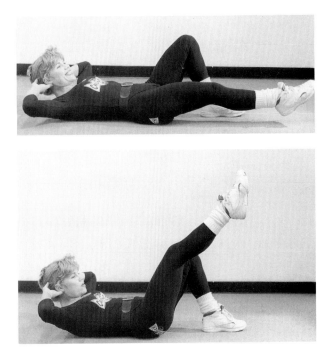

2. Double Crunches

Lie on your back with your knees bent, feet flat on the ground, and hands behind your ears. Use your ABs to simultaneously raise your shoulders and pelvis off the floor. Hold the contraction at the top of the movement for a count. As you lift, exhale and inhale as you release.

Recommendations: Same as Exercise 1.

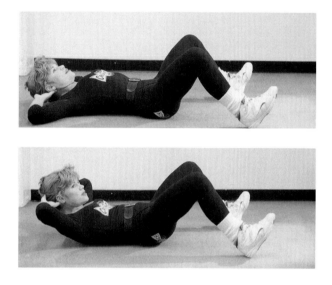

3. Oblique Crunches (page 159)

Recommendations: Do as many repetitions as feel comfortable for three sets.

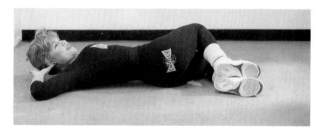

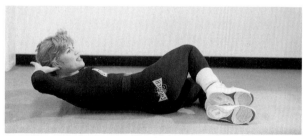

Note on Recommendations for First Two Trimesters: The following recommendations are suggestions, not goals. Stay within your comfort zone. This is especially true during the settling period of the first trimester. During the second trimester, you will feel a bit stronger, and you will probably be able to finish the recommended sets and reps. After the fifth month, most doctors suggest you no longer stay on your back.

Third Trimester

During the end of the second trimester and the beginning of the third trimester, use the following exercises.

4. Back Curls

You can do this exercise on all fours, standing with your back against a wall, or in the fetal position. From these positions, exhale as you curl your back, bringing your chest and pelvis together. Hold the contraction for three seconds (try to exhale) as you try to keep your

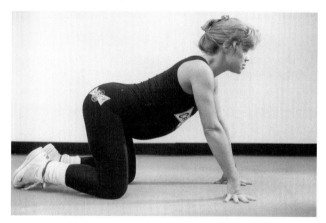

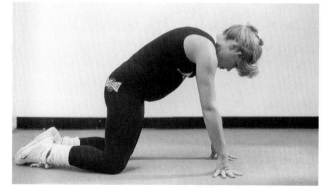

stomach muscles tight. Inhale as you release back to the starting position.

Recommendations: Try to do three sets in each position. Do as many repetitions as feel comfortable.

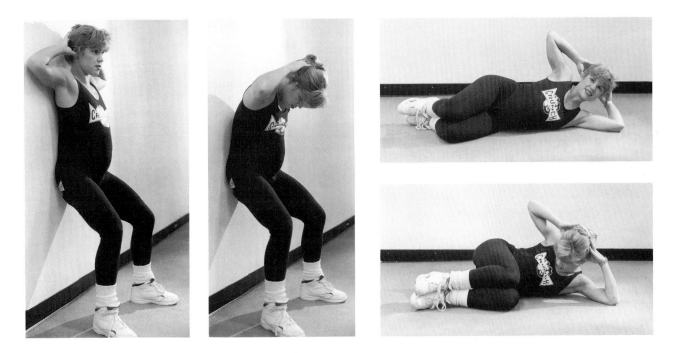

5. Seated Crosses

Sit in a chair with your right leg crossed over your left, forming a triangle between your legs, and place your left hand behind your ear. From this position, cross your left shoulder to your right knee. Exhale as you contract, and inhale as you release and return to starting position.

Recommendations: Start with repetitions of eight to each side and work up to sixteen. Hold the last rep on each set for ten seconds. Try to exhale during the hold. Then switch sides and repeat.

Good luck with your baby, and stay strong!

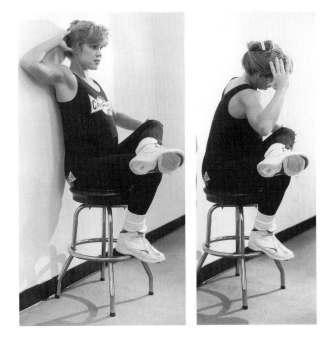

The Time Routines: One-, Two-, and Three-Minute Workouts, by Brett Brungardt

Brett Brungardt is on the Board of Directors of Strength Advantage, Inc., a fitness consultation firm that advises professional and college athletes, coaches, and corporations in the design of fitness programs and state-of-the-art facilities.

INTRODUCTION This routine will give you a quick ABs workout when time is of the essence. One minute during a commercial break is better than nothing.

THE ROUTINES AND EXERCISES

One-Minute Combo Exercise

1. **Reverse Crunches** (page 86) to **Crunches: Knees Up with a Twist,** alternating sides (page 158), to **Crunches: Legs Straight Up** (page 131).

The exercises are performed in the sequence listed. After Reverse Crunches, the knees and feet are elevated to the proper starting position for the Cross Crunches. Then legs are elevated to the straight-up position for the final exercise of the sequence. These three exercises done in succession constitute one repetition. Do as many reps as you can in one minute without a breakdown in technique.

Two-Minute Routine

1. **Bent-Leg Hip Raises** (page 90)	15 reps
2. **Crunches with a Twist** (page 158)	15 reps
3. **Toe Touches: V Spread** (page 161)	15 reps
4. **Crunches: Knees Up** (page 130)	15 reps

Three-Minute Routine

1. **Hip Raises** (page 88)	15 reps
2. **Reverse Crunches** (page 86)	15 reps
3. **Elbow to Knees: Double-Leg Cross** (page 155)	20 reps
4. **Crunches: Frog Legs** (page 134)	20 reps

Senior ABs by Debbie Holmes

Debbie Holmes is the coordinator for the adult fitness program at San Diego State University. She is also the founder of Holmes Personal Training, which provides in-home training in the San Diego area.

ABDOMINAL CONCERNS FOR THE ELDERLY In most cases, there are very limited concerns associated with the elderly population. However, as the body ages, there are a few prevention concerns that become important when performing any exercise program. When working with the older population, all contraindicated exercises should be avoided. Contraindicated exercises are those exercises that place undue stress on any part of the body. Knees and hips are the most susceptible areas for these kinds of exercises.

When working the abdominal area, you'll need to refrain from exercises that do not support the lower back and exercises that put undue stress on hips, elbows, or shoulders. For instance, abdominals done from a decline bench, which begin sitting upright and then dropping back for a half-sit-up, do not provide adequate support for the lower back. Other examples are those exercises that require a forced twist from the lower body (i.e., holding knees to one side while doing crunches for obliques). And lower abdominal work, which requires being on your elbows, should also be limited.

In order to assure safety for your older population, it may be advisable to concentrate on duration of exercise instead of intensity. Encourage seniors toward increased numbers of repetitions instead of increasing the difficulty levels of the exercises.

SUGGESTED EXERCISES FOR THE OLDER POPULATION Begin lying on back with knees hugged into chest. Slowly release knees, keeping low back on the floor, letting your feet rest flat on the floor.

1. Crunches: Knees Up (elbows behind the head or crossed on chest) (page 130)
These can be varied a number of ways:
Keep stomach tight, avoid any extra rocking

Beginners:	10–20 crunches
Intermediate:	20–40 crunches
Advanced:	50+ crunches

2. Crossovers (Ankle supported on opposite knee) (page 144)
Curl up opposite elbow to supported knee, one side at a time

Beginners:	10–20 crunches
Intermediate:	20–40 crunches
Advanced:	50+ crunches

3. Crunches: Knee Bent with a Twist (Both knees up with ankles lifted off the floor) (page 157)
Curl opposite elbow to opposite knee, alternate right and left

Beginners:	10 to each side
Intermediate:	25 to each side
Advanced:	50 to each side

4. Reverse Crunches (Both knees up, with hands supporting under hips) (page 86)
Gently pull your knees up to your chest, pull hips off of floor, relax head on floor, concentrate on pulling with stomach

Beginners:	10 reverse crunches
Intermediate:	20 reverse crunches
Advanced:	25+ reverse crunches

5. Oblique Crunches (Gently allow knees to flop over to one side, do not force) (page 114)
Perform straight crunches, concentrating on the ceiling, one side at a time

Beginners:	10–20 crunches
Intermediate:	20–40 crunches
Advanced:	50+ crunches

The Bulls Multicrunch Sports Routine
by Al Vermeil

Al Vermeil is strength and conditioning coach for the Chicago Bulls. Vermeil is the only strength coach to have a World Championship ring from both the NFL and the NBA. He was the former strength coach for the San Francisco 49ers. Al is currently president of Vermeil's Sports and Fitness, Inc., which specializes in athletic and occupational fitness programs. He is also on the cutting edge of new training technology with the development of Vermeil's Time Machine.

THE EXERCISES

Multicrunch Routine

1. Crunches: Legs Straight Up (page 131)	10 reps
2. Crunches: Legs Straight Up, Spread (page 142)	10 reps
3. Crunches: Knees Up (page 130)	10 reps
4. Crunches: Knees Bent (page 129)	10 reps
5. Crunches: Knees Bent, Spread (page 137)	10 reps
6. Crunches: Split Leg (page 136)	10 reps each side
7. Oblique Crunches (page 114)	10 reps each side

ABS WISDOM
- When you choose a routine, you need to know your purpose. For example, a weight lifter needs thick ABs to protect the back. Most people don't need this mass in their ABs.
- Make sure you mix up and change your routine.
- In this field, we share our knowledge, and Charlie Francis was a big influence in this routine.

The Ice Routine
by Dave Smith

Dave Smith is the strength and conditioning coach for the New York Rangers.

ABS WISDOM
- When you exercise your ABs, you want to be sure to maintain a balance between your obliques and your rectus abdominis.
- When you exercise, you want to isolate the AB muscles and not recruit other muscles to help do the work.
- Signs of cheating are: feet coming off the ground, hands pulling on head or coming off the chest, rocking in the hips.
- When you're exercising, the goal is to fatigue the muscles with the minimum amount of work.
- Do one set of each exercise until you have a breakdown in technique.

THE EXERCISES
1. **Crunches: Knees Bent.** Come up as high as you can, while still keeping your lower back on the floor. (page 129)
2. **Crunches: Knees Bent with a Twist (Oblique Catch).** There is a slight variation on the twist in this movement. You want to have your arms in the extended position, and as you cross your shoulder toward your opposite knee, stretch both hands to the outside of the knee. as if you are reaching to catch a pass. (page 157)
3. **Foot Drags:** Start with your hands under your buttocks and chin to chest. From this position, you are going to drag your heels to your butt, keeping constant tension on the lower ABs. This exercise can also be done with a partner holding your feet and giving resistance as you drag your heels toward your buttocks.
4. **Standing Twists:** With light weights extended in front of you. (page 119)

The Soho Routine
by Lidija Houck

Lidija Houck is the founder of Soho Fitness Center, one of the oldest one-on-one training centers in New York City. Her clientele is a Who's Who of the world's top models, actresses, and artists.

THE EXERCISES
1. Hanging Knee Raises (page 99)	3 sets of 10 to 15 reps
2. Leg Raises (page 95)	3 sets of 10 to 15 reps
3. Side Knee-ups (page 173)	3 sets of 10 to 15 reps
4. Crunches: Knees Bent (page 129)	3 sets of 10 to 15 reps

ABS WISDOM
- Consciously contract on each repetition.
- Don't arch your back.
- Practice contracting your ABs throughout the day when you are standing.
- Change your routine often. Don't get stuck doing the same exercises in the same order over and over again.

The Tom Platz Routine
by Tom Platz

Tom Platz is the legendary "Golden Eagle." He is a multi-Mr. Universe and holder of many other top bodybuilding titles, and has had many face-to-face showdowns with Arnold Schwarzenegger, his erstwhile rival. Schwarzenegger has stated, "You have to understand Tom has pushed his body beyond what was previously thought possible. He is really something else."

After twelve years in California, Platz has settled in Stamford, Connecticut, to take on a new role, talent coordinator of the World Bodybuilding Federation (WBF), a new division of Titan-Sports, Inc. He has recruited the most elite and exciting bodybuilders in the world as the nucleus of the new organization.

ABS WISDOM

The Basics
- AB work is no different from work on any other body part.
  1. You have to isolate the muscle.
  2. You have to contract and extend the muscle.

The Mind
- The most important element in AB training is the mind-muscle link:
  1. You must bring the mind to the muscle.
  2. Mentally feel the contraction in every rep.
  3. Enter the muscle with your mind.
- You could do everything else wrong, but if your mind is in the right place, concentrated and focused, your ABs will improve. And you can't train your ABs and have good development if you don't have the mental power and focus. This may sound extreme, but you cannot underestimate the power of the mind. There are a lot of *AB*less scientists who know in theory how to make muscle grow, and there are a lot of athletes who know exercise science and don't get results. You have to connect the mind to the muscle, put the mind in the muscle and feel the contraction and extension in every rep, just as you do in a dumbbell curl.

Instinct
- The second most important element is instinct.
- You have to do the exercises that feel right for you.
- You need to develop the ability to listen to your body. Everyone is different, and ultimately you are the only one who can find the right path for development.

Education I do not want to deny the place of education. To find the best way, you must exhaust all resources. You need to know your body type and your genetics. For example, I used to train ABs with Frank Zane. We'd get on the Roman Chair, and I'd be fatigued after about twenty repetitions, while Zane could keep going for ten minutes. This is because Frank has predominantly Red fibers, which are better for long-duration activities. And I have predominantly White fibers, which are more explosive but fatigue quicker. What feels right will usually be right. Intellectual choices must stay close to your instincts. For me, I had to take my strong genetic body part out of the movement. In my case, it was my legs. They would always get involved in my AB work. To counteract this, Roman Chair sit-ups became the core of my routine, along with side bends, twists, and isometrics. My body position in the Roman Chair limits my leg involvement. The routine that follows is what has worked best for me. It may take some personal experimentation (trial and error). But in any routine, there will be exercises and concepts you benefit from, especially if you have a similar body type.

THE ROUTINE

1. **Roman Chair Sit-ups:** Work up to three sets of maximum repetitions (to failure). When you can't do any more, finish up with an isometric squeeze. Remember that the quality of the repetitions is what's important. So if you can do only eight reps, stay with quality and work your way up. Position yourself on the front edge of the Roman Chair, so your legs just act as hooks holding you in position but are not activated. (page 178)
2. **Side Bends:** Ten minutes. (page 116)
3. **Twists:** Ten minutes. (page 119)

On both these exercises work up to the ten-minute goal.

4. **Isometric Leg Raises:** Three to five isometric sets. Hold for a ten count.

Description: Lie on a bench and raise your legs and hips off the bench. This position is similar to a shoulder stand. But don't use your arms to push and hold yourself up. Use your stomach muscles. Your legs will naturally want to fall down. Keep them up and squeeze a peak contraction into the ABs for a count of ten.

Note: Rest no longer than a minute between sets. As your condition improves, rest less.

The Mr. Olympia AB Routine by Tony Pearson

Tony Pearson is an elite professional bodybuilder and winner of the "Best ABs" in the Mr. Olympia Contest.

ABS WISDOM

- It is important to know your genetic strengths and weaknesses.
- The quality of each repetition is key:
  1. Stay flexed throughout the entire range of motion.
  2. Squeeze out a contraction at the top of each movement.
- Be patient. Don't expect to see results for two to three months.
- I work them every day in a pre-competition phase.
- Off-season I work them every other day.
- It's also important to work the ABs for health reasons:
  1. Improves posture and gives your lower back support.
  2. Improves balance.
  3. Helps prevent injury in other lifts (squatting, for example).

THE ROUTINE

1. **Hanging Leg Raises:** 4 sets, 15 to 20 reps. 2 sets up to 90-degree angle and 2 sets with feet-to-face level (page 102).
Alternative: Leg Raises off a Bench: 4 sets of 20 (page 95).
2. **Cable Crunches:** 4 sets, 15 to 20 reps (page 141).
TIP: Keep weight shifted over your knees. Bring head down to your knees.
3. **Crunches with a Twist:** 4 sets of 20 on each side. Complete a set of 20 on one side, then a set of 20 on the other side (page 157).
TIP: Don't alternate from side to side; give muscles a chance to rest.

MORE ABS WISDOM

- I recommend doing Pyramid sets on each exercise using light weights. Start out with a warm-up set using no weight and progressively add weight with each set.
- Rest no longer than sixty seconds between sets.

NOTE: This is an advanced routine from an elite bodybuilder. Work up to the recommended sets and repetitions gradually.

The Corporate Routine by John Buzzerio

John Buzzerio is the fitness supervisor for New York Health and Racquet Clubs. He trains the fitness instructors for all locations. John specializes in corporate fitness planning. He is available for private consultations in the areas of business management, exercise programming, and club design. John is a member of the American College of Sports Medicine and has special certificates as an exercise test technologist, exercise specialist, and program director. John has a B.A. in physical education and a master's in exercise physiology.

ABS WISDOM I have been training corporate executives, ranging from commodity traders to CEOs, and they all want the same thing—the best abdominal exercise to trim their stomachs. Unfortunately, there is not one best exercise for everybody. There are too many variables involved. The two exercises in this routine are chosen for the executive whose time is premium. Most executives come in the club and have twenty to thirty minutes to work out. This means they come in and do a quick circuit. The following two exercises work the major stomach areas and can be used as a warm-up or warm-down.

THE EXERCISES

1. **Crunches: Knees Bent** (page 129)
2. **Standing Twists** (page 119)

To achieve the best results, you need to focus your mind on your ABs and see the muscles working. This will give you the best results in the least amount of time. I would recommend working up to 30 reps for crunches and a minute of standing twists.

The Golf Routine
by Brett Brungardt

Days 1 and 3

1. **Seated Knee Raises** (page 94)   20 reps
2. **Standing Twists** (page 119)   50 reps, turning both directions for one repetition
3. **Knee-ups: Double Leg Cross** (page 168)   20 reps, turning both directions for one repetition
4. **Crunches: Split Leg** (page 136)   30 reps each leg
5. **Crunches: Knees Bent with a Twist** (page 157)   30 reps, turning both directions for one repetition
6. **Modified Jackknives** (page 111)   30 reps
7. **Back Extensions** (see below)   15 reps

Day 2

1. **Seated Knee Raises** (page 94)   3 sets of 10 reps with a light weight held at the ankles
2. **Russian Twists on a Roman Chair** (page 163)   3 sets of 15 reps each way
3. **Side Leg Raises** (page 109)   3 sets of 20 reps using isometric contraction 10 seconds every tenth rep
4. **Side Crunches** (page 114)   3 sets of 20 reps using isometric contraction 10 seconds every tenth rep
5. **Crunches: Knees Up** (page 130)   3 sets of 20 reps, weighted
6. **Toe Touches** (page 132)   3 sets of 20 reps, weighted
7. **Back Extensions**   3 sets of 10 reps, weighted. See Lower Back chapter for an exercise that fills your back needs and fitness level.

- Program to be performed three times a week. To be preceded by a warm-up. Days 1 and 3 are to be performed with no rest between sets. Day 2 is to be performed with thirty seconds' rest between sets. Take a day off between workouts.
- The Golf Abdominal routine has three main goals: First, to gain strength, endurance, and flexibility in midsection. Second, to improve power initiation and power transference through the midsection. And finally, to improve trunk and hip rotational power and flexibility.

The Three-Way Crunch
by Marty Stajduhar

Marty Stajduhar is strength coach for the Texas Rangers. He is also a physical therapist and director of Dallas Sports Rehabilitation Center. Marty was a catcher and third baseman in the Oakland A's organization. He has his master's degree in physical education from Arizona State University. He lives with his wife, Lisa, and children Nikolas and Adriana.

Multicrunch: With medicine ball on top of bench

Purpose: To facilitate muscle contractions in the abdominals, buttocks, and lower back

Starting Positions: These positions are in order of difficulty.

Level 1 Starting Position: Lie flat on your back, knees bent, upper calves resting on ball, knees bent at a 90-degree angle, and hands in position of choice.

Level 2 Starting Position: Lie flat on your back, knees bent, lower calves resting on ball, knees bent at a 90-degree angle, and hands in position of choice.

Level 3 Starting Position: Lie flat on your back, knees bent, ankles resting on ball, knees bent at a 90-degree angle, and hands in position of choice.

Movement: Lift your hips off the floor by tightening your AB muscles (one to two inches only), and keep your knees bent at a 90-degree angle. Then perform a standard crunch movement, lifting your shoulder blades off the floor.

Routine: Start at Level 1 and work up to three sets of 30 to Level 3.

TIPS
- Balance your legs lightly on the ball.
- The balanced position may initially cause the exerciser to roll to one side or another in an attempt to maintain balance.
- Keep your thighs perpendicular to your body in all positions.

The Lower Back Routine
by Mike Brungardt

INTRODUCTION This routine is specifically designed for those with lower-back problems. I have had great success in using this routine in conjunction with lower-back exercises to alleviate chronic lower-back problems: setting clients back on their feet and doing the activities they enjoy without pain. But everybody is different, so you should check with a medical professional before beginning this program.

1st Two Weeks

1. **Modified Knee Raises: Single Leg** (other leg elevated at 90 degrees)—
   Week 1: 2 sets × 10 reps each leg (page 93)
   Week 2: 2 reps × 15 reps each leg
2. **Crunches: Knees Up** (hold at top)—
   Week 1: 10 reps
   Week 2: 15 reps (page 130)
3. **Crunches: Knees Bent** (legs in air)—
   Week 1: 3 sets × 10 reps
   Week 2: 3 sets × 15 reps (page 129)

   Week 1: 30 sec. rest between sets
   Week 2: 15 sec. rest between sets

Weeks 3 and 4

1. **Modified Knee Raises** (both legs)—
   Week 3: 2 sets × 15 reps
   Week 4: 2 sets × 20 reps (page 93)
2. **Crunches: Knees Bent** (hold at top)—
   Week 3: 2 sets × 15 reps
   Week 4: 2 sets × 20 reps (page 129)
3. **Toe Touches** (mid)—
   Week 3: 3 sets × 15 reps
   Week 4: 3 sets × 20 reps (page 132)

Weeks 5 and 6

1. **Reverse Crunches**—20, rest 10 sec.; 20 no rest (page 86)
2. **Crossovers**—20 each side, no rest (page 144)
3. **Crunches: Knees Up**—20, no rest (page 130)
4. **Toe Touches** (fast)—20, rest 10 sec.; 20, rest 10 sec.; 20 (page 132)

Weeks 7 and 8

1. **Bent-Leg Hip Raises**—10 reps (page 90)
2. **Knee Raises**—10, rest 10 sec.; 10 (page 91)
3. **Reverse Crunches**—10, rest 10 sec.; 10 (page 86)
4. **Crossovers**—20 each side, rest 10 sec.; 20 each side (page 144)
5. **Crunches: Knees Bent**—20, rest 10 sec.; 20 (page 129)
6. **Crunches: Knees Up**—20, rest 10 sec.; 20, rest 10 sec.; 20 (page 130)

Weeks 9 and 10

1. **Bent-Leg Hip Raises**—10, rest 10 sec.; 10 (page 90)
2. **Knee Raises**—10, rest 10 sec.; 10, no rest (page 91)
3. **Reverse Crunches**—10, rest 10 sec.; 10 (page 86)
4. **Crossovers** (foot on knee)—20 each side, rest 10 sec.; 20 each side (page 144)
5. **Crunches: Knees Bent** (hold at top)—20, rest 10 sec.; 20 no rest (page 129)
6. **Toe Touches** (fast)—20, rest 10 sec.; 20, rest 10 sec.; 20 no rest (page 132)
7. **Medicine Ball Reverse Crunches** (5 lb.)—30 sec., no rest (page 86)
8. **Medicine Ball Leg Overs: Bent Knee, Double Leg** (5 lb.)—30 sec., no rest (page 123)
9. **Medicine Ball Crunches: Knees Up** (5 lb.)—30 sec., no rest (page 130)

Weeks 11 and 12

1. Incline Bent Leg Hip Raises—10, rest 10 sec.; 10 (page 90)

2. Incline Knee Raises—10, rest 10 sec.; 10 (page 91)

3. Reverse Crunches—10, rest 10 sec.; 10 (page 86)

4. Crossovers (foot on knee)—20 each side, rest 10 sec.; 20 each side (page 144)

5. Crunches: Knees Bent (hold at top)—20, rest 10 sec.; 20 no rest (page 129)

6. Toe Touches—20, rest 10 sec.; 20., rest 10 sec.; 20 no rest (page 132)

7. Medicine Ball Reverse Crunches (8–10 lb.)—1 min., no rest (page 86)

8. Medicine Ball Leg Overs: Bent Knee, Double Leg (8–10 lb.)—1 min., no rest (page 123)

9. Medicine Ball Toe Touches (5–10 lb.)—1 min. (page 132)

The Olympic Ski Routine
by Mike Brungardt

INTRODUCTION This routine was designed for former Olympian and current professional skier Beth Madsen. If you are an avid skier and would like to utilize this routine, I suggest that you build up to it by going through "The System" in this book.

THE ROUTINE

1. Hanging Leg Raises—10, rest 10 sec. (page 106)

2. Hanging Knee Raises—10, 10 sec. rest (page 99)

3. Incline Leg Raises (Incline Knees to Chest with 10-lb. medicine ball)—10 (page 95)

4. Incline Knee Raises with 10-lb. medicine ball—10 (page 93)

5. Knee-ups—30, rest 10 sec.; 30, no rest (page 167)

6. Crossovers—20 each side, rest 10 sec., 20 each side (page 144)

7. Toe Touches: with a Cross—20 each side, no rest (page 160)

8. Crunches: Knees Bent (Hold at Top)—30 (page 129)

9. Toe Touches—3 sets, 50 reps, rest 10 sec.; 50, rest 10 sec.; 50 (page 132)

10. Medicine Ball Reverse Crunches (10 lb.)—1 min. (page 86)

11. Medicine Ball Leg Overs: Bent Knee, Double Leg (10 lb.)—1 min. (page 123)

12. Medicine Ball Toe Touches (10 lbs.)—1 min. (page 132)

ABS WISDOM Abdominal strength for skiers is extremely important in assisting them to keep their upper torso parallel to the fall line. Strong ABs also protect the lower back, which is extremely important if you are skiing the bumps. In previous seasons, Beth had always experienced lower-back pain, but when she utilized this routine, she experienced no back pain the entire season.

The Cowboy Circuit Routine
by Mike Woicik

Mike Woicik is strength and conditioning coach for the Dallas Cowboys.

ABS WISDOM
• We do a lot of different circuits.
• Usually, these circuits are made up of six to eight exercises done back-to-back.
• We do ABs four times a week off-season and twice a week in-season. But this varies from player to player.
• It is important to have variety in your ABs routine. This can be done in a number of ways. A couple of examples of ways to create variety are: Vary the length of your isometric holds at the finish of your movements and vary the speed of your movement. Do one set fast, one set slow. Do one repetition fast, one repetition slow, etc. The combinations are endless.
• We also use the AB Flexor Machine, by FLEX, extensively. This is the best piece of equipment I have ever seen to work your lower ABs.

• What follows are just a couple of examples of routines we do. The repetition scheme, of course, will depend on your fitness level.

ROUTINE ONE: CIRCUIT
1. **Crunches: Knees Bent** (hands on hips)—20 reps (page 129)
2. **Crunches: Knees Up** (hands behind ears)—20 reps (page 130)
3. **Toe Touches**—20 reps (page 132)
4. **Crunches with a Twist: Knees Up**—20 reps (page 157)
5. **Leg Raises with Movement Sequences:** Crisscrosses—50 reps. Hold at 6 inches off the floor (page 97)
6. **Reverse Crunches**—10 to 15 reps (page 86)
7. **Leg Raises**—5 seconds up and 5 seconds down, 10 reps (page 95)
8. **Side Crunches:** Roman Chair: 15 reps on each side (page 114)

ROUTINE TWO: BREAKDOWN
Ideally, this routine should be done with the AB Flexor Machine and Nautilus Crunch machine. If you don't have access to these machines, substitute Bent-Leg Hip Raises (making sure to roll your hips off the floor with each repetition) and Crunches (with legs in position of choice).

1. **AB Flexor Machine** or **Bent-Leg Knee Raises**—20 reps
2. **Nautilus Crunch Machine** or **Crunches**—20 reps
   Following this order, decrease repetitions by five reps, for each exercise, on each consecutive set. So your rep scheme for each exercise will be twenty, fifteen, ten, five, for a total of four sets and a total of a hundred reps. Increase weight resistance as needed.

The Sports Enhancement Routine by Greg Brittenham

Greg Brittenham is strength and conditioning coach for the New York Knickerbockers. He has been instrumental in the design and implementation of performance enhancement programs for a variety of sports, including several top-ten (in the world) tennis players, teams and individuals of the National Football League, baseball's National League, the United States Gymnastic Federation, and World Champion Cyclists, to name a few. He is currently in the final stages of producing a comprehensive videotape and accompanying training manual geared toward developing strength and power in the abdominals and low back.

STRENGTHENING THE ABDOMINALS FOR IMPROVED SPORTS PERFORMANCE AND INJURY PREVENTION

Training Guidelines

• Start with one set of four to six repetitions on each exercise. As strength levels improve, increase the number of repetitions per set, and gradually increase the number of sets per session. Never sacrifice form for added sets and repetitions.
• Try to maintain a "tight" abdominal contraction throughout the set. Keep rest to a minimum between sets, and never rest between exercises *during* a set.
• Always fatigue the "weaker" abdominal muscles first. Therefore, the order with which to maximize abdominal strength should be: 1) obliques; 2) lower ABs; and 3) upper ABs. Because the upper abdominals assist with movements in the lower and oblique abdominal region, it is important *not* to fatigue the upper ABs first, thereby decreasing the amount of work performed by the other muscles of the trunk and torso.
• Avoid exercises that place the spine in an arched position (i.e., straight leg sit-ups, Roman chair, etc.).
• Keep workouts balanced. Always train opposing muscle groups (e.g., low back) equally to prevent muscle imbalances.

ABDOMINAL TRAINING PROGRAM

INITIAL PHASE
(APPROXIMATELY 3–4 WEEKS)
4–6 REPETITIONS   1 SET

TRAINING PHASE

(2 WEEKS EACH)	REPETITIONS	SETS
I	8	1
II	10	1
III	12	1
IV	6	2
V	8	2
VI	10	2
VII	12	2
VIII	6	3
IX	8	3
X	10	3
XI	12	3

NOTE: Athlete should perform one *complete* circuit of each exercise, rest one to two minutes, and begin second circuit. Always follow an abdominal training session with a comprehensive cool-down/flexibility routine, including several low back contraction exercises.

THE EXERCISES

1. **Side Crunches: Straight Legs** (legs extended straight out) (page 114)
   Hold for a two count in "up" position. Switch sides.
2. **Oblique Crunches** (page 159)
   Hold for a two count in "up" position. Switch sides.
3. **Crunches: Frog Legs** (page 134)
   Hold for a two count. Touch shoulder blades and repeat.
4. **Sit-ups: Knees Bent** (arms extended) (page 174)
   Hold for two seconds and go down slowly.
5. **Crossovers** (page 144)
   Hold for a two count. Shoulder blades should touch on "down." Perform one complete set, and then repeat with right leg over left leg.
6. **Sit-ups: Feet Up** (page 176)
   Hold for a two count. Maintain hip and knee flexion throughout the exercise.
7. **Toe Touches** (page 132)
8. **Bicycles** (page 145)

The Intermediate Routine by Steven Schultz

Steven Schultz is the strength and conditioning coach at Stanford University, where he is in charge of creating and administering the strength and conditioning programs for all of the sports at Stanford. He is also cofounder of FlexIt, a private fitness consulting firm in Mountain View, California. Steven has his M. Ed. in exercise physiology from the University of Nebraska.

THE EXERCISES

1. **Hanging Leg Raises** (page 102): to fatigue
2. **Hanging Knee Raises** (page 99): to fatigue
3. **Crossovers** (page 144): 20 on each side
4. **Side Crunches** (page 114): 20 on each side
5. **Crunches: Legs Straight Out** (page 133): 20 reps
6. **Crunches: Legs Straight Up** (page 131): 20 reps

Don't rest between exercises.

Tennis and Auto Racing Routines by Jim Landis

Jim Landis has been a personal trainer for twelve years. He specializes in strength conditioning. He works with business executives, television personalities, and professional athletes. He trains such top Indy car drivers as Danny Sullivan and Emerson Fittipaldi, tennis champions Chris Evert, Martina Navratilova, and Pam Shriver, and Olympic gold-medalist ice skater Scott Hamilton, to name a few. Jim has worked with the Arizona Heart Institute and the Aspen Institute for Fitness and Sports Medicine, and he is a member of the National Strength and Conditioning Association.

TENNIS Abdominals for the game of tennis are essential because of the dynamic nature of the sport. Tennis requires not only good balance development and muscular strength, but also a high degree of muscle endurance. For instance, there is a very great force applied from the legs to the arms in the tennis serve, as well as during the powerful rotation during ground strokes. In Martina's and Chrissie's programs, we include not only low-intensity basic abdominal exercises, but also some advanced strength-building movements. Their easiest exercises are usually performed on the floor and done with short rests between sets (two sets of twenty reps being the norm). This light routine usually includes the following exercises:

THE EXERCISES

	SETS	REPS
1. Reverse Crunches (page 86)	2	20
2. Double Crunches (page 146)	2	20
3. Side Jackknives (page 112)	2	20
4. Toe Touches (page 132)	2	20
5. Bicycles (page 145)	2	20

Rest between sets ten to twenty seconds.

The routine they use to develop more strength would include the following exercises, using only two to three of the options for the day. The intensity is so much higher in this series of exercises that the reps will fall between eight and fifteen in two to three sets. This routine includes:

1. Hanging Leg Raises (page 102)
2. Sit-ups: Roman Chair (page 115)
3. Russian Twists (page 162)
4. Leg-overs: Double Leg (page 124)
5. Side Bends—Standing with Dumbbells (page 117)
6. Rotary Torso Machine (See machine chapter)

With any layoff from working out, Martina and Chrissie will usually do a week or two of the lighter routine before including the more advanced exercises. They usually include abdominals three days per week, often alternating light and heavy routines.

AUTO RACING For car racing, abdominal strength and endurance help to keep the driver in proper alignment in the car during the tremendous forces incurred during the turns (sometimes they pull three to four g's countless times in a race) and driving over relatively rough surfaces at speeds in excess of 200 mph. Obviously, strength becomes critical in maintaining control over the car. Drivers have an off-

season of several months at which time Danny and Emerson take this opportunity to increase their basic strength. Their light routine would look much like Martina's and Chrissie's. Their heavy routine would include many of the same exercises. The main difference is the constant demand on the drivers where endurance of the abdominals becomes most important, as races often continue for two or more hours. Therefore, their routines often include supersets, or circuit routines. Some of these routines include:

1. Reverse Crunches (page 86; to **Seated Leg Raises** page 95)
2. Hanging Leg Raises (page 106; to **Sit-ups: Feet Up** page 176)

Light-day floor exercises with five seconds or less rest between sets. Circuit routines include:

1. Hanging Leg Raises to **Sit-Ups: Feet Up** to **Reverse Crunches** (page 102; page 176; page 86)
2. Rotary Torso Machine (See machine chapter.) to **Reverse Crunches** to **Crunches: Knees Up** (page 86; page 130)
3. Russian Twists to **Incline Sit-Ups** to **Bicycles** (page 162; page 179; page 145)

Understanding Your Individual Body Imbalance by Kirk Rivera

Kirk Rivera is a continuing-education provider for the American Council on Exercise, and he is the author of *Strictly Abdominals*. His unique motivational style contributes to the certification of fitness professionals internationally. His motivational contributions were an important part of chapters 17 and 18.

STRENGTH Every "body" has imbalances—there is no such thing as true symmetry. You probably know without too much thought which one of your arms is stronger than the other, right? Well, the same strength imbalance exists in your abdominals: Let's find out why.

STRETCH Flexibility in the hip flexors and quadriceps directly affects the degree of flexibility in the abdomen.

COORDINATION Are you right-handed or left-handed? Don't think for a second that this dramatic difference in your basic everyday movement won't affect how well you perform abdominally from one side to the next.

The following "Awareness" exercises will help you better understand your IBI, or Individual Body Imbalance.

• Which leg would you kick a ball with?

Whatever your answer, that leg has a tighter hip flexor and quadricep. You can expect this side of your *lower* abdomen to be stronger at first, but then it will seem to lose mobility as it approaches fatigue. A simple Lunge Stretch can determine just how much mobility you have to start with.

• If you were coming home with an arm-load of groceries, which leg would you use to hold open the door?

Whatever your answer, that leg and lower abdomen are more coordinated than the other. You can expect a cleaner, more exacting performance from this side. Don't expect the other to behave as fluidly.

• You are reaching high to screw in a lightbulb. On which leg is your weight, and with what arm are you reaching?

Whatever your answer, the leg your weight is on is your body's supporting leg. *Your hamstring and gluteus will be tighter here.* Any exercise demanding flexibility there will be fighting against your basic structure. The arm you're reaching with is your coordinated side. This side will be doing all the best work. You're going to have to show some patience for your weaker, less coordinated sides.

Also . . .

There are no hard and fast rules . . .

Your body is your body. It is a great asset for anyone to start a coordinated program (and abdominal programs are coordinated programs) with a sense of where he is and what he can expect. All this is an effort to *keep your performance frustrations from becoming unsafe.*

The Martial Arts Routine by Stephen Rittersporn

Stephen Rittersporn is a second degree black belt in Shorin Ryu karate and a black belt in jujitsu. He has been practicing martial arts for fifteen years. He teaches classes and gives private instruction in self-defense and the martial arts.

THE ROUTINE
1. **Knee Raises** (page 91)
2. **Leg Raises with movement variations** (page 95)
   A. Criss-Crosses
   B. Kicks
3. **Standing Twists** (page 119)
4. **Side Bends Without Weight** (page 116)
5. **Leg Overs: Double Leg** (page 124)
6. **Russian Twists** (page 162)
7. **Crossovers** (page 144)
8. **Crunches: Knees Bent** (page 129)

Repetitions and Sets: Start out by doing 10 reps per exercise for one set and work up to 20 reps per exercise for three sets. Gradually decrease your rest time.

ABS WISDOM
• Always warm up before you workout.
• Work your ABs in isolation, it's safer.
• Keep your lower back pressed against the floor whenever possible.
• Oblique work is important for martial arts, because kicks and throws involve a lot of rotary motion.
• Strong ABs are also important for absorbing blows and protecting internal organs.
• Don't kill yourself. Take it slow.

The Hawkeye Routine
by Dan Gable

Dan Gable is head wrestling coach at the University of Iowa. During his career he has racked up nine consecutive NCAA championships and a career total of eleven, creating one of the greatest dynasties in college athletics. He was the Olympic coach for the 1980 and 1984 teams and Olympic gold medalist in the 1972 games, where he was named the best-conditioned athlete in the world.

EXERCISES AND ROUTINE
1. Bent-Leg Hip Raises (page 90)
2. Leg Raises: Crisscrosses (page 97)
3. Leg Raises: Kicks (page 97)
4. Full Sit-Ups with a Twist (page 175)
5. Crunches, Knees Up (page 130)
6. Body Punches: One person tightens his ABs and the other person lightly punches the area for a thirty-second period.
CAUTION: Be careful when doing this exercise; the goal is to tone the ABs, not to injure the other person.

Do each exercise to fatigue.

ABS WISDOM
- I train my wrestlers from the top of their head to the tip of their toes.
- Self-massage is a good way to warm up an area before you work it.
- I stress total body conditioning, but leg and AB strength is particularly important. Most techniques involve driving off the legs, and lifting and twisting movements for throws. AB strength and endurance is very important in these movements.

Club Body Tech Routine
by Donna Cyrus

Donna Cyrus is director of aerobics at Miami Beach's most popular fitness club, Club Body Tech. Her experience—twelve years of teaching aerobics and fitness classes—has been intensified by her background of dancing on Broadway in *A Chorus Line* and *Grease*.

Donna teaches a half-hour "Abdominals Only" class every day at Club Body Tech, basing her instruction on one important belief: that the optimal way to work abdominals lies in understanding the breathing process. Many people hold their breath when working out, not realizing how important oxygen is to proper muscle development. What follows are Donna's basics from Club Body Tech's famous "Abdominals Only" class.

This technique is vital to all AB exercises:
Lie down and press the lower back into the floor. Put both feet flat on the floor while flexing knees. Expand abdominal muscle with air. Put one hand on stomach and press air out of abdominal muscle, much like letting the air out of a balloon. Once this idea is grasped, then go on to the following exercises.

UPPER ABDOMINALS
1. Keeping the same position as above, grasp both hands behind neck and crunch forward while expelling air and pulling ABs into the lower back. Do 10 times *slowly*.
2. Keeping the same position, twist left elbow to the right knee, trying to touch the elbow to the knee 10 times *slowly*. Repeat with right elbow and left knee.
3. Bring both knees to the elbows 10 times. This works the upper abdominals.

LOWER ABDOMINALS
1. Keep feet above knees. Press arms into the floor next to your waist and *slowly* bring knees upward toward upper body while lifting hips off the floor (10 times).
2. Extend feet to ceiling and press hips off the floor (10 times).

OBLIQUES (SIDE ABDOMINALS)

1. Take knees to the right while keeping torso centered. Clasp hands behind the neck and lift shoulders off the ground while aiming chin to the ceiling (10 times). Repeat 10 times with knees to the left.

This basic routine is excellent for total abdominal conditioning and should be expanded by adding to the number of repetitions as your proficiency increases. One major way to improve the workout is to *add music!* Select tunes with a steady beat, slow enough to practice the breathing technique described earlier. Start the routine doing 1 repetition per beat, then halfway through do *2* repetitions per beat, that is, double-time!

Lower AB Blast
by Kurt Brungardt

This routine is designed to attack a problem area for both men and women—the lower ABs. The exercises are ordered in decreasing difficulty, so the most difficult exercise comes first and the easiest comes last.

1. Hanging Leg Raises: Straight Leg (page 102)
2. Hanging Leg Raise: Bent Leg (page 103)
3. Reverse Crunches on Incline Board (page 87)
4. Hip Raises (page 88)
5. Bench Reverse Crunches (page 87)
6. Reverse Crunches (page 86)

GUIDELINES
• Work up to 20 reps on each exercise.
• Take short rests between exercises.
• Since the exercises are ordered in decreasing difficulty, it is like taking weight off a bar (or picking up a lighter set of dumbbells) and continuing to exercise.

On The Slant
by Kurt Brungardt

A slant board uses gravity to add resistance. This routine takes advantage of gravity from two different angles, giving you a simple and intense workout by alternating two exercises. Most slant boards are adjustable, so increase the angle as you get stronger.

THE ROUTINE

First Set

1. Reverse Crunches (page 86): 20 reps
2. Crunches with a Cross (page 158): 20 reps

Second Set

1. Reverse Crunches: 15 reps
2. Crunches with a Cross: 15 reps

Third Set

1. Reverse Crunches: 10 reps
2. Crunches with a Cross: 10 reps

GUIDELINES
• Do not rest between exercises or sets unless needed.
• Increase repetitions as needed, maintaining the five rep intervals.
• You can also add sets, going all the way down to five reps or resting then doing the entire sequence over again.

Left to Right
by Kurt Brungardt

This fast and furious routine hits all three stomach areas with each exercise. It is intended for advanced exercises.

THE ROUTINE
1. Elbow to Knees: Double-Leg Cross (page 155)
2. Leg Scissors Crunch with a Cross (page 170)
3. Elbows to Knees: Bent-Knee Cross (page 153)

GUIDELINES

- Start out with 20 repetitions for each exercise (ten on each side) and work up to 40 reps (20 on each side).
- Just take a brief pause between exercises.
- If you need to rest, keep reducing the rest time with each workout.
- When this gets easy take a one minute rest and do another set. Work up to three sets.

Going Ballistic
by Kurt Brungardt

This routine is designed for advanced exercisers. The exercises have an extended range of motion and also place emphasis on other muscles, such as the hip flexors. These muscles are used in similar ways in many sports. It is important that your body is fully warmed up, making this a good routine to do at the end of your workout.

ROUTINE

1. **Side Knee-ups** (page 173)
2. **V-ups** (page 171)
3. **Body Tuck** (page 180)

GUIDELINES

- Work up to 30 reps for each exercise.
- Rest as needed.

Circles
by Kurt Brungardt

This routine uses two exercises to target the three AB areas.

THE ROUTINE

1. **Circles** (page 148)
2. **Reverse Crunch Circles** (page 149)

GUIDELINES

- Complete 20 reps of each exercises without resting between the exercises (this equals one set).
- Rest 30 seconds, then do your second set.
- Work up to five sets.

Bench Blaster Circuit Routine
by Kurt Brungardt

This routine uses a basic bench to increase the intensity in a circuit of five exercises. Having to maintain balance on the bench also works important stabilization muscles.

THE ROUTINE

Lower ABs

1. **Bench Hip Raises** (page 89): 30 reps
2. **Bench Reverse Crunches** (page 87): 30 reps

Obliques

Make sure your shoulder blades drop off the edge of the bench for these exercises (the same way they do in a Bench Crunch).

3. **Crossovers** (page 144): 30 reps (15 each side)
4. **Catches** (pinch the outside of the bench with your feet for stability if needed): 30 reps (15 each side)

Upper ABs

5. **Bench Crunches** (pinch the outside of the bench with your feet for stability if needed) (page 86): 30 reps

GUIDELINES

- Do one circuit resting as little as possible between exercises.
- You can build on this routine by adding circuits: rest between 1 and 3 minutes between circuits. Work up to three circuits.

21 Breakdowns

This routine attacks the ABs from opposite ends while also targeting the lower and upper obliques. This routine is designed for the advanced exerciser.

THE ROUTINE

First Set

1. **Corkscrews** (page 147): 21 reps
2. **Crunches: Legs Straight Up** (page 131): 21 reps

Second Set

1. **Corkscrews:** 18 reps
2. **Crunches: Legs Straight Up:** 18 reps

Third Set

1. **Corkscrews:** 15 reps
2. **Crunches: Legs Straight Up:** 15 reps

Fourth Set

1. **Corkscrews:** 12 reps
2. **Crunches: Legs Straight Up:** 12 reps

Fifth Set

1. **Corkscrews:** 9 reps
2. **Crunches: Legs Straight Up:** 9 reps

Sixth Set

1. **Corkscrews:** 6 reps
2. **Crunches: Legs Straight Up:** 6 reps

Seventh Set

1. **Corkscrews:** 3 reps
2. **Crunches: Legs Straight Up:** 3 reps

GUIDELINES
- Do not rest between exercises unless needed.
- Keep rest time between sets to a minimum (under thirty seconds). Eventually, do the entire routine without resting.

Frontline Fitness 3D Middle Muscle Routine by Liz Neporent, M.A., C.S.C.S.

Liz Neporent is the president of Frontline Fitness, a New York–based fitness consulting company that specializes in programming, facility design, and management. She is the author of *Fitness for Dummies, Weight Training for Dummies, Buns of Steel*, and *Abs of Steel*. And she is a contributing editor for *Good Housekeeping* and *Shape*.

INTRODUCTION This routine includes exercises that isolate the rectus, obliques, and lower-back muscles, plus exercises that work several muscles at once. Stretches help balance middle-body strength and flexibility. Beginners can do one set of the first exercise in each category.

ROUTINE

Rectus

1. **Crunches: Knees Bent** (page 129)
   1–2 sets   8–15 reps
2. **Reverse Crunches** (page 86)
   1–2 sets   8–15 reps

Obliques

1. **Bicycles** (page 145)
   1–2 sets   8–15 reps (each direction)
2. **Circles** (page 148)
   1–2 sets   8–15 reps (each direction)

Lower Back

1. Opposite Arm and Leg (on Stomach) (page 52)
        1–2 sets   8–15 reps (each side)
2. Basic Trunk Extension (page 53)
        1–2 sets   8–15 reps

Stabilization and Multi-Muscle Movements

1. Rolling Ball: gently roll up and down your spine through the range of motion illustraed in the following pictures.
    1–2 sets   8–15 reps (balance on the top of your sit bones at the completion of each repetition)

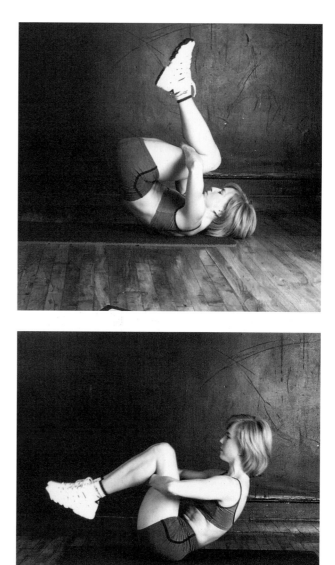

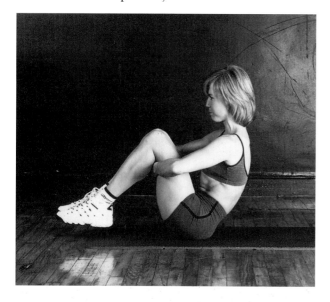

2. Body Tuck
    1–2 sets   8–15 reps (roll your body up to the tuck position, then roll it back down to the starting position)

Stretches

1. Back and Stomach (page 61)
    1–2 sets   20–60 second hold
2. Knee-to-Chest Hug (page 60)
    1–2 sets   30–60 second hold

Mr. California Routine
by Steven Wilde

Steven Wilde is a boxer, personal trainer, and former competitive bodybuilder. He lives in Los Angeles.

THE ROUTINE
This routine is designed to work all your core muscles (ABs, hip flexors, and lower back) and add size to your abdominal area.

1. Full Sit-ups (page 174)

2. Hanging Leg Raises with a Cross (both legs) (page 184)

GUIDELINES
• Work up to five sets of each exercise.
• Work up to 25 reps for each exercise.
• Eventually add weight to increase intensity for Full Sit-ups. When you add weight you'll need a partner to hold your legs down.
• Rest three minutes between sets.

CHAPTER TWENTY

Creating Your Own Routine

by BRETT BRUNGARDT

The time will come when you have to leave the nest and create your own routine. This may cause anxiety, and that's expected. Don't worry, this chapter will give you the tools you need to design your own routine, so you can become your own personal trainer.

Part One: The Design Model

When creating an AB routine, you need a basic design model or blueprint to work from. You can think of the ABs as four separate boxes that comprise three areas: Area One (Lower ABs), Area Two (Obliques), and Area Three (Upper ABs).

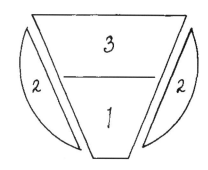

To build a routine, you need to think about how you want to shape and strengthen each area or box. This will depend on your individual needs and goals: weak areas, the look you want, sports-specific training, etc. It is always important, however, to keep muscle balance in mind.

Since the exercises in this book are categorized according to the three basic AB areas, you'll find it easy to plug in exercises and personalize your routine.

Part Two: Basic Concepts

The following are key principles (along with the principles in Chapter 3) you need to consider when building your routine.

ENERGY SYSTEMS
Exercises are not all created equal. To ensure the best overall abdominal development, you'll need to include three kinds: Exercises of high intensity and short duration, exercises of medium intensity and medium duration, and exercises of low intensity and longer duration should all be in your training regimen. In other words, you need to include exercises that are difficult and wear you out quickly, and exercises that are easier, allowing you to do them for longer durations. Programming these different kinds of exercises into your routines is a way to create variety and train for specific sports and activities. Being aware of energy output is a way to intelligently incorporate both endurance and strength training into your regimen. This is done in the last level of the system.

Muscle Balance: The exercises you choose should work all the muscle groups in the abdominal area (see anatomy) at a variety of angles.

Never completely neglect one abdominal area to work weaker areas. If you have strong areas, still train these areas but not as intensely as the weak areas. This means choosing exercises of less intensity, doing fewer reps, using fewer exercises for that area, or any combination of the above.

Muscle balance is a key consideration when choosing exercises. The abdominal muscles work together during most activities. They also play an important role in supportive and structural alignment. When one muscle, or muscle group, becomes considerably stronger than others, the potential for injury is greatly increased.

SPECIFICITY
Exercises should be chosen to fit your specific needs, for example:

Training Stage: Exercise choice will be affected by your training stage: a pre-conditioning stage, a maintenance stage, a peak performance stage, etc.

Sport or Activity: The specific needs of your sport are a major consideration in exercise selection. You need to train for specific kinds of movements as well as the type of energy output used in the sport.

Personal Goals: When choosing exercises, you have to be aware of your specific goals: what you want and how much time you are willing to spend. If you are a bodybuilder, your goals are going to be much different from someone who wants to firm up a little and improve his or her posture.

EXERCISE ORDER
In general, the best order for exercises is from largest to smallest. But the order can also be affected by individual goals and the need for variety. If your primary goal is to shape your obliques, then you will want to target them first. But staying with the same exercise order for extended periods of time will cause complacency (no adaptation), which means less than optimal gains.

VOLUME
Volume as it relates to abdominal strength training can be described as total number of repetitions and the number of sessions per day, week, month, etc. When creating a progressive series of routines, you want to keep an eye on total volume, making sure you're doing enough but not too much. Volume is also important as it relates to intensity. When intensity increases, volume should decrease.

INTENSITY
Intensity relates to the difficulty of an exercise, resistance (weights), if any, and amount of rest time.

Variation: Variation is the most neglected training principle. Training needs to be varied for the following reasons: to prevent overtraining, to avoid training plateaus, and to alleviate the boredom of monotonous training.

Variation is related to intensity and volume. When you first started working your ABs, it was easier to shock your muscles and cause adaptation. As you become more advanced, you will need to change your workouts more frequently. An example of how to do this is to choose exercises of greater difficulty that will naturally decrease your repetitions (volume), while increasing your intensity. Another way to create variety is to do the opposite: increase repetitions and decrease your intensity. When you're considering variations in volume and intensity, you may want to vary similar training days within a training week. You will have a day of high-intensity training (heavy) and one of low-intensity training (light). The terms "heavy" and "light" days can be misnomers. To obtain the optimal training effect, overload (i.e., muscle failure) should always occur—on both "heavy" and "light" days.

Part Three: Periodization

Periodization is a systematic and progressive training method designed to aid in planning and organization. This cyclical training encompasses all the basic training principles and helps bring performance to a peak. It is utilized by the greatest athletes and strength coaches in the world (many of whom are included in this book).

The scope of this book does not allow for a detailed treatment of periodization, but the following summary will help you in creating your abdominal routines. The basis for periodization was the General Adaptation Syndrome (GAS), developed during the 1930s. It was intended to describe a person's ability to adapt to stress. The three distinct phases of adaptation, according to the GAS, are:

Alarm Stage: This relates to the individual's initial response to training. This could result in a temporary drop in performance due to stiffness and soreness.

Resistance Stage: This is when the exerciser adapts to the training stimulus by making gains in strength, tone, and endurance.

Overtraining Stage: If stress placed upon the exerciser is too great, then the following can happen:

• Plateauing and a decreased performance level
• Chronic fatigue
• Loss of appetite
• Loss of body weight, or lean body mass
• Increased illness potential
• Increased injury potential
• Decreased motivation and low self-esteem

During this stage, the desired training adaptations are not likely to occur. Outside stresses—for example, social life, nutrition, amount of sleep, work, etc., also need to be considered to avoid overtraining.

The goal then is to remain in the resistance stage of training, where your body is making the compensations to the stresses applied and continually improving. This is where the concepts of periodization apply.

The Cycles

Once your goals have been defined, the next step is planning, which can be divided into four training phases. Before going into these cycles, you will need a definition of the peaking period, which is the goal of all these cycles.

THE PEAKING PERIOD

This is the period where all your training culminates, bringing out the best possible results. This will, of course, be different for everybody, depending on individual goals. For the elite athlete, this can be very complicated, because several variables have to come together at once: strength, endurance, specific-sports skill, diet, mental state, etc. The same is true for a bodybuilder. Things become simplified if it's just the stomach you're concerned about. But even then, things aren't that simple. If you want your ABs to peak out for a vacation on the beach, you should be focusing on three variables: your AB routine, diet, and cardiovascular work. Again, the peaking period is when you bring all these elements together at their highest level.

MACROCYCLE

The macrocycle is the longest of the training phases. Its length varies from one individual to another, depending on the goals. In general, the macrocycle lasts from the end of one peaking period to the beginning of the next peaking period. The macrocycle defines long-term goals and a specific time frame in which you want to peak: six weeks, six months, or one year. The macrocycle contains three components: preparation (mesocycles and microcycles), peaking, and transition.

MESOCYCLE

The next-largest phase is the mesocycle. Mesocycles make up a macrocycle. The number, length, and purpose of your mesocycles will depend on the goals of your macrocycle. A mesocycle is a phase that has specific goals. For example, the goal of the first mesocycle may be that of preparation, which might include high volume and fairly low intensity training to build a base of strength. The next mesocycle's goals might include an increase in intensity (more difficult exercises, shorter rest periods, etc.) while maintaining volume requirements to build strength and endurance. The next mesocycle goal may be oriented for strength gains (increase in intensity, increase in resistance, sets, rest time, lower volume). The final mesocycle, in which you reach peak condition might include more intensive evaluation: What areas are weak and need extra work; what areas are strong; what has worked best in the past; diet, mental state, etc. Peaking for abdominals will differ from peaking for sports performance. Training intensity and volume may continue to increase when you're bringing your ABs to a peak. When peaking for sport performance, they decrease, allowing for rest and recuperation before the event. The better the preparation—that is, the better your condition—the longer you will be able to maintain your peak.

MICROCYCLE

Within each mesocycle are smaller units called "microcycles." Microcycles further refine the objectives by manipulating training variables on a daily basis.

One day might include training of high volume (reps) and moderate intensity, while the next day may include training of high intensity and moderate volume (reps). Or it may become even more complex, as in our ultimate ABs section (see Chapter 18), which works different muscle groups and changes intensity levels from day to day.

TRANSITION

Unfortunately, maintaining peak anything for a long period of time can be very difficult. The cycle following a peaking period is the transition phase. The abdominals can maintain a peak longer than most muscle groups. So the possibility exists when training the ABs to have more frequent and longer peaking periods. This is not to say that your ABs can't look great all the time. And the concepts of the transition phase will help ensure this.

A transition phase allows for regeneration and recuperation, both mentally and physically. It also introduces variety into the program. The transition phase allows you to start at a higher training level in the next macrocycle. Without a transition phase the rigors of peaking will ultimately lead us into stage three of the GAS: overtraining. The body needs time off from the peaking phase, with its diet restrictions and the high intensity of training. The transition phase allows the right amount of recovery so you jump right back to a growth phase.

When most people think of recuperation, they think of sitting on their butts and doing nothing. With the transition phase, this is not true. You continue to train, but at lower volumes and intensities. Substitute activities you like. Have fun! Do light abdominal work once to twice a week. No more than sixty repetitions per day should be undertaken.

Using the design model in part one of this chapter and following the basic concepts outlined here and in Chapter 3, you can choose exercises from the book and create your own customized routine. Then, following the natural cycles of periodization, you can create a series of progressive routines, staying as long as possible in the growth and peaking phases, to achieve the ABs you want.

A CASE STUDY

For example, if you wanted to peak for a vacation in Hawaii during the first week of March and it is now the beginning of December, you would plan a three-month macrocycle.

You would probably want to break this down into one-month mesocycles with two-week microcycles for the first two months, and one-week microcycles for the last month, as you prepare to peak.

Your breakdown may go something like this:

First month: This would be your preparation period. You would build a safe foundation doing low-intensity exercises with high reps. During your two microcycles, you would gradually decrease your rest time.

Second Month: During this period, you would add exercises and increase the intensity of your exercises. You would use your two-week microcycles to accomplish these goals. The goal of the first microcycle would be to add one new exercise per area. In the second microcycle, you would replace certain exercises with more difficult ones.

Third Month: During this cycle, you start to change your workouts more often, going to one-week microcycles. You may have a heavy week, adding isometric holds, followed by a week of high repetitions with no rest between sets. This could be followed by a week where you mix your light and heavy days. And during the last microcycle, you would train every day in preparation for peaking out for that first day on the beach. During this week, you may train more instinctively, switching your workout every day and training weak areas.

Also, during this week all other facets of your training must peak (diet, cardiovascular, and strength training).

Good luck with your advanced principles. The applications of these principles will lead to your ultimate success and longevity in training.

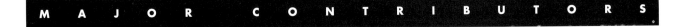
Brett Brungardt is on the board of directors of Strength Advantage, Inc., a fitness consultation firm that advises professional and college athletes, coaches, and corporations in designing fitness programs and facilities. Brett is the coauthor of *The Strength Kit*, a manual for planning strength and conditioning programs for all levels: scholastic, collegiate, and professional.

He is also a professor of exercise science at Colorado Mountain College. He is the author of numerous publications in the area of fitness. He has an M.Ed. in exercise science from the University of Houston and is a member of the National Strength and Conditioning Association.

Mike Brungardt is on the board of directors of Strength Advantage, Inc. As a member of Strength Advantage, he has given seminars at clinics for fitness educators in schools and health clubs throughout the country. Along with Brett Brungardt, he developed the strength program for the San Antonio Spurs. He has worked with such professional athletes as ski racer Beth Madsen (1990 Rookie of the Year). He specializes in the mental and motivational aspects of sports performance and is also coauthor of *The Strength Kit*. He has also been involved in the consulting and design of a wide range of fitness facilities.

Mike graduated from Central State University of Oklahoma, where he wrestled and played baseball. He has nine years of coaching experience at Northwest High School, in Grand Island, Nebraska, one of the most successful athletic programs in the state of Nebraska during the eighties.

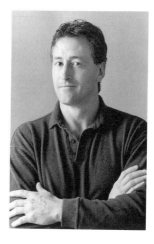

Becky Chase is a registered dietitian. She currently maintains a private practice through her business, Alpine Nutritional Services. Becky specializes in sports nutrition and eating disorders. She consults through the Aspen Club and MidValley Sports Medicine and Fitness Clinic, Inc. Becky lectures regularly to students and consumer groups about nutrition and programs she has developed: Market Smarts (a grocery-store tour) and *Stop Dieting, Start Thriving* (a program for compulsive eaters).

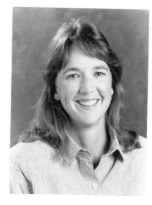

Becky has written many articles for newspapers, magazines, and hospital publications. She is currently working on a book based on her Market Smarts program. Becky has a B.S. and an M.S. in clinical dietetics from Texas Woman's University.

Bryon Holmes is director of programs for Muscular Skeletal Evaluation and Rehabilitation at the University of California San Diego, Department of Orthopedics. As a member of the Holmes Personal Training team, he also does private fitness consultation for individuals and corporations. Bryon specializes in preventive care and rehabilitation of the lower back. He is a member of the American College of Sports Medicine. Bryon has a B.S. and an M.S. in exercise physiology from the University of Florida.

Debbie Holmes is the coordinator for the adult fitness program at San Diego State University. She is also the founder of Holmes Personal Training, which pro-

vides in-home training in the San Diego area. She is a member of the American College of Sports Medicine and I.D.E.A. She has her B.S. and M.S. in health science and education from the University of Florida and she is the founder of *The Living Well News Letter.*

Dave Johnson is a writer and personal trainer in New York City. He was assistant strength coach at Wake Forest University. He holds a B.A. in writing from Wake Forest and an M.F.A. in writing from Columbia University.

Soho Fitness Center for letting me use its state-of-the-art facility to photograph exercises. Special thanks to Mitch Zoleman, the new owner, whose fitness expertise is always helpful and who makes Soho Fitness Center one of the best places in New York to train.

Crunch Fitness Centers for donating clothing.

Lights, Camera, Flex Modeling and Talent Agency for loaning me Joe and Rick. Definitely the place to go if you're looking for athletically fit men and women.

Mayfair Hotel Baglioni put up my brother and loaned us gym equipment for the photo shoot.

Eugenie Tartell, P.C. Upper West Side Chiropractic Center. Thanks for giving your expertise on issues involving the lower back and for the chiropractic care you've given me.

Lance Winn created the original designs for the anatomy illustrations. Lance is a painter, poet, and recent graduate of Rhode Island School of Design. Again, who said it's hard to work with artists?

Joan Erskine, M.A., of the Diet/Exercise Connection in Brooklyn, gave her support and advice in the beginning stages of this book. Her commitment to helping people improve the quality of their lives through exercise is inspiring.

Denny Bonewitz, the assistant strength coach at the University of New Mexico, gave his expert advice in developing routines.

Andrew Brucker is a New York photographer. He specializes in portraits and nudes. His work has appeared in numerous art journals, magazines, and books, including *Interview, Details, Rolling Stone, New York Woman,* and *Männer-Vogue,* to name a few.

THE MODELS

Lisa Alexander is an actress and model. She has studied at HB Studio and has a B.A. in theater/communications from the State University of New York. She has been in numerous films, videos, and television commercials.

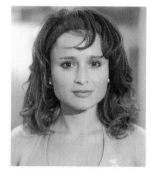

Alfonso Berry is a personal trainer and competitive bodybuilder. His accomplishments include: Natural World Cup Championships, Natural Eastern U.S.A., Eastern Classic Championships (teenage division). Alfonso is a personal trainer at New York Health & Racquet Club and he is also pursuing a career in acting and modeling.

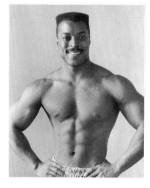

Susan Bernstein is senior staff nurse in Recovery at St. Vincent's Hospital in New York City. She competed in gymnastics for eight years and is the captain of her volleyball team in the Urban Professional League.

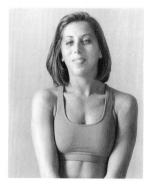

Mike Brungardt (see bio in major contributors).

Greg Brittenham

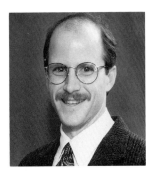

Jim Buzzerio

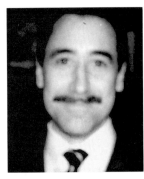

Cameron Dougan

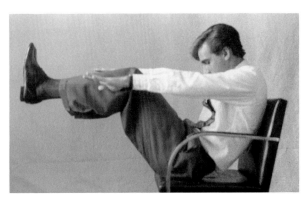

Jim Fantone is an actor and personal trainer. He is a graduate of the New York Academy of Dramatic Arts and performed with its third-year company. Jim was in the U.S. Army, where his specialization was as a master fitness trainer.

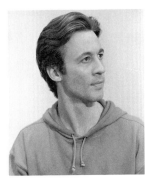

Joe Finfera is an all-natural competitive body-builder. He specializes in body photography. He has also appeared in numerous stage, television, and video productions. Courtesy of Lights, Camera, Flex.

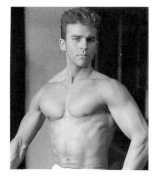

John Guidera is a model and workout enthusiast. He has appeared in numerous print and television ads.

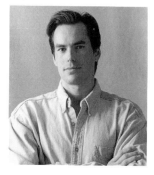

Rick Huegli

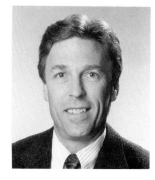

Dave Johnson (see bio in major contributors).

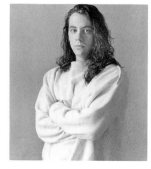

Jim Landis

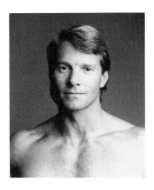

Jeff Laughlan is a personal trainer at Plus One Fitness Clinic. He has a B.S. degree in both exercise physiology and diet and nutrition from Kansas State University. He is also a member of the New York Athletic Club rowing team.

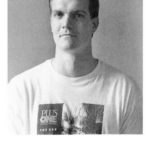

Robin Mandel-Naylon

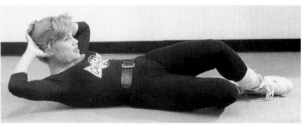

Jeff Martin

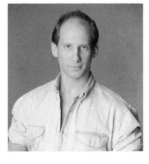

Mike Motta

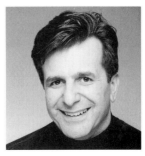

Tom Platz

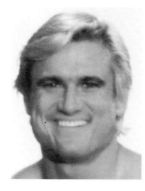

Stephen Rittersporn

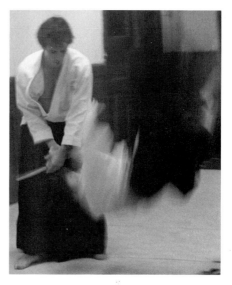

Rick Rivera is an all-natural bodybuilder. He placed second in the New York's Finest Bodybuilding Competition. He has been a policeman for three years. And he is just breaking into a career in modeling and acting. Courtesy of Lights, Camera, Flex.

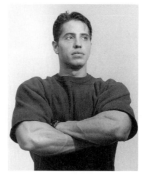

Jeff Rockford is a personal trainer and owner of Washington Square One to One, a fitness center that specializes in one-on-one training.

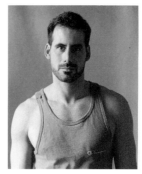

Julie Seyfert is finishing her Ph.D. in developmental psychology at Columbia University. She is also an avid rock climber, skier, roller-blader, backpacker, and world traveler. She has also appeared in numerous television and print ads.

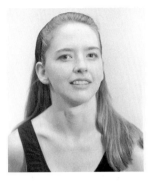

Steven Schultz

Jessica Yates is a writer and artist. She went to school at Bennington and Vassar College.

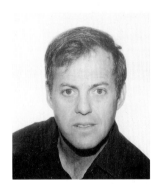

Al Vermeil

INDEX

About the Author

Kurt Brungardt has been a personal trainer in New York for seven years. He has trained a wide range of individuals: Olympic and professional athletes, celebrities, Wall Street executives, and senior citizens. He is a member of Strength Advantage, Inc. He created and hosted the bestselling video *Abs of Steel for Men*.

He grew up in Kansas, was an NCAA intercollegiate wrestler, and now lives in New York City.

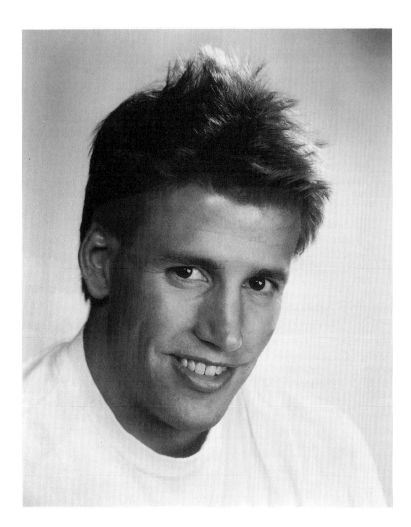

THE BEST IN FITNESS BOOKS FROM VILLARD

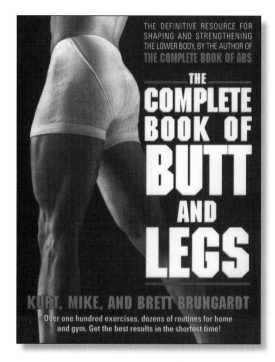

THE COMPLETE BOOK OF BUTT AND LEGS

Kurt, Mike, and Brett Brungardt

0-679-75481-4
292 pages
$20.00/$24.95 Canada

The definitive guide to strengthening and toning the lower body.

THE MARINE CORPS BASIC TRAINING WORKOUT

Coming in January 1999

U.S. Marine Corps

0-375-75132-7
144 pages
$19.95/$27.95 Canada

The fundamental, no-frills workout and complete fitness program, written with the full cooperation and participation of the U.S. Marine Corps.

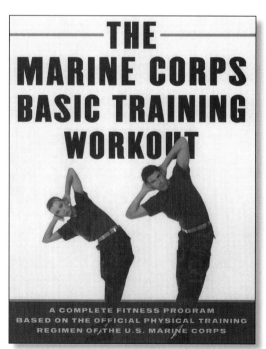

VILLARD